VAGUS NERVE

Mastering and Understanding Polyvagal Theory. Daily Exercises and Massages Stimulations Will Help You to Reduce Anxiety, Panic Attacks, Depression, Inflammation, Anger, and Chronic Illness.

© Copyright 2020 - All rights reserved.

The content contained within this book may not be reproduced, duplicated, or transmitted without direct written permission from the author or the publisher.

Under no circumstances will any blame or legal responsibility be held against the publisher, or author, for any damages, reparation, or monetary loss due to the information contained within this book. Either directly or indirectly.

Legal Notice:

This book is copyright protected. This book is only for personal use. You cannot amend, distribute, sell, use, quote or paraphrase any part, or the content within this book, without the consent of the author or publisher.

Disclaimer Notice:

Please note the information contained within this document is for educational and entertainment purposes only. All effort has been executed to present accurate, up to date, and reliable, complete information. No warranties of any kind are declared or implied. Readers acknowledge that the author is not engaging in the rendering of legal, financial, medical, or professional advice. The content within this book has been derived from various sources. Please consult a licensed professional before attempting any techniques outlined in this book.

By reading this document, the reader agrees that under no circumstances is the author responsible for any losses, direct or indirect, which are incurred as a result of the use of the information contained within this document, including, but not limited to, errors, omissions, or inaccuracies.

TABLE OF CONTENTS

Introduction 1
Chapter 1: What Is The Vagus Nerve? 7
Chapter 2: Activating The Vagus Nerve 15
Chapter 3: Benefits 23
Chapter 4: Inflammation And Autoimmune Diseases.... 35
Chapter 5: Vagus Nerve Malfunctions 49
Chapter 6: Polyvagal World 59
Chapter 7: Polyvagal And Autism 65
Chapter 8: Vagus Nerve And Anxiety Disorder 73
Chapter 9: Understanding Anxiety, Ptsd, Trauma And Depression 85
Chapter 10: Causes Of Anxiety, Depression, And Inflammation 95
Chapter 11: Power Of Your Body With Self-Help Exercises And Techniques 109
Chapter 12: Music 135
Chapter 13: Social Media 139
Chapter 14: Create Safety 143
Chapter 15: Meditation To Activate The Vagus Nerve .. 145
Chapter 16: Yoga Treatments For Vagus Nerve 164
Chapter 17: Exercises To Balance The Vagus Nerve 168
Chapter 18: Activating Your Vagus Nerve Effortlessly .. 190
Chapter 19: More Activities And Exercises To Trigger Your Vagus Nerve 201
Chapter 20: Vagus Never Healing With Natural Body Exercises 218
Chapter 21: Practical Exercises To Stimulate The Vagus Nerve 224
Chapter 22: Window Of Tolerance 256

Chapter 23: Body And Mind Connection 266
Chapter 24: How Pain, Stress And Anxiety Affect Your Life
.... 270
Conclusion 280

INTRODUCTION

The vagus nerve comes from a Latin name "Vaga" and is considered to be a wandering nerve much like a vagabond would wander; thus, some may call it the vagabond nerve. It is also known as the "wandering nerve" because it has multiple branches that diverge from two thick stems rooted in the cerebellum and brainstem that wander to the lowest viscera of your abdomen, touching your heart and most major organs along the way.

The vagus nerve is fantastic for preventing inflammation. Having a small amount of inflammation during illness is quite alright, but when it gets out of hand, it is often then linked with a number of conditions such as arthritis. When the vagus nerve gets a signal to say that there is inflammation in the body due to there being cytokines present in the body, the vagus nerve will then respond quickly to the brain in order to activate its anti-inflammatory neurotransmitters in order to allow the body's immune system to regulate.

The vagus nerve is also incredibly well-known for

helping your brain to develop memories! Studies were done with rats in a University in Virginia that showed that stimulating the vagus nerves of these rats had greatly strengthened their memories. This is due to a neurotransmitter called norepinephrine, which gets released into the amygdala of the brain where memories are formed and thrive. Other studies that had been done on humans had also found incredible results with regards to a future treatment for conditions such as Alzheimer's disease as well as dementia.

The vagus nerve is also known to assist with the body's need to breathe. A neurotransmitter called acetylcholine that is created by the vagus nerve is what gets triggered in order to let your lungs know that now is a good time to inhale and exhale for the sake of survival. Did you know that this is also why the use of Botox in any cosmetic types of surgeries can be potentially dangerous to your overall health? This is because the use of Botox is known to mess with the production of the acetylcholine neurotransmitter, which in turn would prevent you from being able to breathe. On the bright side, though, this is where the power gets put in your own hands with stimulating breathing exercises that can help you to strengthen your vagus nerve by yourself.

The neurotransmitter called acetylcholine was the first-ever neurotransmitter discovered by scientists and got its name originally from a physiologist named Otto Leowi, who learned of the substance through causing a reduction in heart rate during a vagus nerve study. He called the substance 'Vagusstoff,' which is directly translated from German for "vagus substance."

Much like how the vagus nerve is very intimately related to your lungs, it is equally related to your heart. Using specific electrical impulses through to the heart muscles, the vagus nerve can control your heart rate somewhat like a pacemaker. Doctors will generally use this information by measuring your heart rate variability between your individual heartbeats over time in order to know whether anything may be wrong with your ticker. To do this, they work very closely with the vagus nerve.

The vagus nerve is completely responsible for keeping up with your body's relaxation response. As the vagus nerve is the part of your body that creates the neurotransmitter acetylcholine, it is what is responsible for getting your body to calm down when your sympathetic nervous system has a 'freak out' moment and releases adrenaline and cortisol into your blood. By having the tendrils of the vagus nerve connected to each of your vital organs, your body is able to release the proteins and enzymes needed to relax you, such as prolactin, oxytocin, and vasopressin.

A person is more likely to have a speedy recovery from illness, injury, or stress when they have a strengthened vagus nerve. They are able to strengthen their vagus nerve through any of the techniques that we have mentioned in this book.

Your vagus nerve acts as a walkie-talkie between your digestive system and your brain. Electrical impulses are sent between your gut and your brain to tell you whether you may be feeling nauseous, sore, or even to tell you that something is making you nervous or anxious. You shouldn't ignore your "gut feelings." They are often right and know what is best for you and your body!

Just as we discussed earlier, fun fact: overstimulation of your vagus nerve is by far the most common cause of a person fainting. If you are feeling faint because of fear such as the fear of needles or blood, it isn't because you're a baby or weak, but because your vagus nerve has been overstimulated in a short span of time and you are now getting what is called 'vagal syncope.' Your body responds to the sudden stress by quite literally turning itself off like a light switch as the blood in your brain is restricted, and you ultimately end up losing consciousness. By lying down or sitting and breathing, you may be able to alleviate the symptoms before you drop.

The vagus nerve has been known to reduce the signs of inflammation through electronic stimulation greatly. Studies were done on rats in order to determine whether stimulation of the vagus nerve would be able to reduce inflammation in the rat, and the results were so successful that the study was moved onto humans with exceptional results, showing that it may inhibit the inflammation altogether. By using a vagus nerve stimulating implant that allowed for the vagus nerve to be stimulated electronically, a drastic reduction in inflammation was shown as well as remission on arthritis which has no true known cure and is often only treated with anti-inflammatory medications.

Scientists and doctors are currently working on replacing medications and high schedule drugs with vagus nerve stimulation devices. Since vagal nerve stimulation has shown such high success in the treatment of epilepsy, inflammation, and depression, a new medical field is known as bioelectric, has come into play as the future of medicine as we know it. With these new studies, scientists and doctors are hoping to be able to treat illness and injury with as few side effects as possible in the long run.

CHAPTER 1
WHAT IS THE VAGUS NERVE?

Did you know that the human body has 12 cranial nerves? Did you know that each "nerve" is actually comprised of two nerves, typically left and right nerve intertwined to make the "one" cranial nerve. And these nerves are the link between your body and the brain? Have you ever wondered how the brain and body "talk" to one another? It is all through these cranial nerves. Some of the nerves are responsible for sharing sensory information, like how something sounds or what it tastes like. This means these nerves need to have the sensory function to interpret the smell of something. But then there are other nerves that "talk" with the muscles and even some glands. These nerves are called "motor functions." And finally, while most have a single function, either sensory or muscle, there are others that operate with both. The Vagus nerve is one such nerve.

To help you understand where a nerve is located, each cranial number is assigned a number represented in Roman numerals, for example, I is one, II is two, etc. The Vagus nerve is the tenth nerve and is called CNX, or Cranial Nerve Ten.

In Latin, the word "vagus" is defined as "wandering." When you understand a bit more about the makeup of this nerve, you will realize that this description is pretty accurate. The Vagus nerve is the longest in the human body, and it does a lot of traveling around and through it. Basically, it moves from the base of your skull to your lower torso. You will learn more about the passage of this nerve later in this chapter.

There are two parts to the sensory functions of this particular nerve:

1. **Visceral**: This is used to describe the "feelings" or sensations in your body's organs.
2. **Somatic:** This term is applied to your physical "feelings," or sensations in the muscles and skin of your body.

Each part of the sensory function is unique. The somatic function gives information regarding the skin from behind the ears. It also shares this information from the ear canal and various parts of the throat. It is also responsible for the visceral information shared to the brain regardings the majority of your digestive tract, heart, lungs, trachea, esophagus, and larynx. Finally, while it is not the primary "player" in the sensations in your tongue, your Vagus nerve does have a small role in how your tongue's root experiences the sensation of taste.

There are three primary motor functions that the Vagus nerve functions with:

1. **Stimulates digestion and the digestive tract.** This involves involuntary contractions in the majority of your intestines, stomach, and esophagus to help food move through the system.

2. **Stimulates your heart.** The primary goal is to massage the muscles of the heart in an effort to lower your resting heart rate.

3. **Stimulates your mouth.** This stimulation includes the soft palate, or the soft area in the back of the roof of your mouth, larynx, and pharynx.

As you can see, this nerve is a fairly powerful player in not just how you feel, but how you experience the world, you are living in. It impacts everything from your brain to your digestion, and so much in between. This means if something "goes wrong," it can have dire consequences to your health and well-being. To check to see if it is in working order, many physicians will first begin with your gag reflex. It is often done with a cotton swab, where the doctor "tickles" both sides in your back throat. This causes most people to gag involuntarily. If not, there may be something wrong with this nerve.

Some of the common problems that occur for your Vagus nerve include:

- **Nerve damage**
- **Gastroparesis**
- **Vasovagal syncope**

Nerve Damage

Because of the extreme length and vast scope of this nerve, there can be a variety of symptoms indicating it has been damaged. Most of the time, the symptom of Vagus nerve damage depends on the location of the damage. Some of the common symptoms include:

- Stomach acid production is decreased
- Blood pressure is abnormal
- Heart rate is unusual
- Ear pain
- Gag reflux is minimal or lost
- Drinking liquids proves to be a problem
- Wheezy or hoarse voice often
- Loss of voice or challenge speaking
- Vomiting or nausea
- Pain or bloating in the abdomen

Gastroparesis

Gastroparesis is another condition that many experts believe is the result of a damaged Vagus nerve. This concerns the contractions of the digestive tract. When the involuntary contractions are not functioning properly, the stomach cannot empty properly. It is a common side effect of vagotomy. This is a procedure that removes some or all of the Vagus nerve. Side effects common to gastroparesis include:

- Blood sugar fluctuations

- Weight loss that is unexplained
- Bloating or bleeding in the abdomen
- Acid reflux
- Feeling full at the beginning of a meal or not having an appetite
- Vomiting or nausea, especially if the vomit contains food that is not digested even hours after eating

What Exactly Are The Causes Of Vagus Nerve Damage?

This particular nerve materials motor nerve impulses on the muscles of the voice box and tongue, receiving sensory desires coming from the organs, ear, and the throat of the chest as well as belly, and also providing visceral nerve impulses to the glands of the throat, abdominal organs, and chest. Female doctor showing healthcare chart to a female patient resting in the hospital bed.

Diabetes

Diabetes is able to result in neuropathy, or maybe nerve damage, to a variety of distinct body parts. A prolonged rise in blood glucose associated with diabetes is able to modify nerve chemistry and harm the blood vessels which support the nerves. In instances where diabetic issues have destroyed the vagus nerve, it is able to result in gastroparesis, a problem whereby the muscles of the stomach, as well as intestine, aren't able to effectively move meals with the gastrointestinal system. Gastroparesis manifests in symptoms including nausea, abdominal bloat, constipation, heartburn, vomiting, stomach spasms, & decreased appetite.

Alcoholism

Chronic alcohol abuse is recognized to damage nerves, a condition called alcohol neuropathy. Alcohol abuse has a dose-related deadly impact on the autonomic nervous system; of that, the vagus nerve is a portion. Abstaining from alcohol is able to overturn the harm to the vagus nerve. Infection, as well as Surgical Complications Vagus nerve injury, is able to happen following top respiratory viral infections. These infections initially involved signs, for example, cough, runny noses, and nasal congestion. Symptoms that persisted in individuals diagnosed with post-viral vagal neuropathy, throat clearing, included cough, or PVVN, vocal fatigue, and difficulty speaking.

The vagus nerve is often damaged during surgery to the small intestine or the stomach. A process known as laparoscopic hemifundoplication, utilized to treat gastric reflux, continues to be connected with vagus nerve injury.

Vasovagal Syncope

During stressful situations, the Vagus nerve can overreact. When this happens, it can dramatically drop your blood pressure and heart rate, because it is responsible for stimulating the various muscles in your heart to slow down the heart rate. This sudden drop can lead to fainting. Some common stressful triggers include:

- Standing for long periods of time
- The intense strain on the body, including while trying to have a bowel movement
- Having blood drawn or seeing blood
- The concern of harm to the body
- Extreme heat and overexposure

CHAPTER 2
ACTIVATING THE VAGUS NERVE

Through breathing exercises, cold blasts, holding a healthy intestine, and some other basic activities, you can tone your vagal pathways. Modern medicine treats specific organs as part of the disease and overlooks the point that your brain plus central nervous system tells you how to proceed.

Your organs often send a status check with the vagus nerve to your brain to report exactly how it all works. It's a street in two ways. If all goes well, your brain will maintain the status quo. If an organ struggles, it can mean even more information for your brain. Your vagus nerve carries the signal to your organs from your brain to slow down until it's time for your body to spring to action.

Inflammation Tension and Fight or Flight Immune Response

Because the vagus nerves are involved in a lot of things, they must work properly. Continue reading to learn how, through vagal toning, you can help your vagus nerve. There is a relationship between respiration and pulse rate, which is modulated by the nerve of the vagus. It is precisely for this reason that regular yoga practice reduces general stress.

Breathing yoga and then breathing guided exercises will calm your heart rate to minimize your blood pressure. Breathing exercises improved overall vagal tone and, in an experimental group, properly handled prehypertension. Slower breathing exercises improved autonomic characteristics in healthy participants in a single study.

It wasn't fast breathing.

That's how quickly your body thinks you're running from predators.

That sets off the alarm bells of your body and causes a response to stress.

Breathing kit for S.O.S. Tries breathing box when you're panicking or about to blow a gasket.

Inhale a four-count.

Keep a count of four.

Exhale a count of four.

Hang on to a count of four.

Repeat until the controls have your hands available.

Trace your finger in the air in a square format the first few times. It'll help you remember when you're frazzled how to get it done.

The gradual development of your respective lungs signals to slow down to your heart, through your whole nervous system. Your vagus nerve connects all these releases and signals acetylcholine, a calming substance that you can use relaxation methods to give yourself a go at any moment. The vagus response, which delays the activation of the sympathetic nervous system, becomes familiar with the chilly tones.

Constant cold blasts reduce indicators of pressure dramatically.

Chilly exposure helped alleviate anxiety and depression symptoms, possibly modulated by the nerve of the vagus. It stimulates digestion by revitalizing the vagal pathways. Due to anxiety, when the digestion of rats slowed down, cold stimulation reactivated the stomach nerves and got the products going again.

It all happened through vagal paths.

Keep your gut happy. Have you ever learned about the axis of the gut? This describes how your digestive system's microorganisms talking to your brain. Your microbiota is the ecosystem of your body and your skin's pleasant bacteria. They usually talk about the germs in your colon and intestines when someone talks about the microbiome.

Because the microbiome research is building up, the medical community is developing more and more approaches that impact the entire body. Investigating the relationship between the microbiome and the spirits is increasing, and interaction between the gut and the mind depends on the vagus nerve-surprise.

Human and animal models research to support the notion that a prosperous microbiome reduces tension and raises your mood. Rodents that supplemented with different probiotic strains reported reductions in anxiety and stress markers, but not in animals whose were cut vagus nerves before experimentation. Researchers see the beneficial effects of probiotics on people's moods.

Good females who have eaten fermented food for four weeks have shown positive changes in brain activity, particularly in the mental components that manage emotions and feelings. Through animal studies and probably from what scientists know about the vagus nerve, you can well believe that the gut-brain communication here occurs in the vagus nerve.

The very first stage to get through when you have an anxious stimulus is the person who addresses interpersonal interaction-oral language, body language, facial firmness, and several other non-verbal signals. When the stimulus is simply too powerful to reason, the fight or flight reaction triggers your brain. If this fails, the most primitive reaction of fear is probably to play the perception frozen.

If you realize that your fear is irrational, you can use protective measures to stop the panic at the very first level and prevent your brain from reacting with fighting or flight.

Let me share a few things that you can do.

Choose relaxing voices.

One of the ways children experience this phenomenon hardwired.

Children are measurably calmed by the prosodic (singing song), which is also known as mothers.

Changing your speech tone also works for adults.

Guided meditations are accompanied by a slow, rhythmic overall tone, whether personally or even registered.

Using the voice as a source of calming coaxes the mind more easily into a relaxed state than a normal chat.

Train your safety indicators You can train your mind to feel safe with some practice.

Protection measures protect your fear and anxiety from kick-in reactions.

One way to do this is to make your place safe or happy while you are calm.

To do this, you imagine you're in a place where you're completely comfortable, contented, and peaceful.

Use as much sensory information as possible? View sights, sounds, smells, and so on.

Practice this specific visualization often.

In this way, if you begin to feel angry or frightened, you can start a safe place without much effort.

If you want it, it's there.

Check for your myelin.

The vagus nerve is myelinated, which could mean it is filled with an extra fat protective layer that isolates it and enables the signals to move efficiently.

If myelin breaks down on any nerve, the nerve does not do the job.

Surgically implanted vagus stimulator

The vaguely implanted nerve triggers the immune system of the body when you fight.

Physicians use this knowledge to treat inflammatory problems, revitalizing the vagus with pharmaceuticals and electricity.

Surgically, physicians place electric vagus nerve stimulators in individuals with severe depression and epilepsy because they dampen the effect of inflammation.

You should tone the vagus nerve of your baby.

Several factors play into the vagal tone of the child. Babies born early, or mothers born during pregnancy who have anxiety and depression, are of low vagal tone.

Don't worry if you go through a few things during pregnancy. You can help to tone the vague ways of your baby with regular connections and loving attention.

Strong showers almost certainly should wait until the junior is old enough to agree.

Infant massage and kangaroo treatment (holding skin-to-skin baby) develop the vagal tone of the babies during infant years.

If your children go beyond childhood, you can use these methods for toning the vagus, such as cold blows and breathing techniques in the bath.

A massage and a few minutes of goosebumps in your bathroom probably deserve to be considered, because the benefits of vagal nerve toning also extend to every major organ in your body and have come back.

CHAPTER 3
BENEFITS

When you practice deep breathing techniques, you are going to benefit in many ways. Of course, the main why that you are going to benefit is by activating and stimulating your vagus nerve. This, of course, means that you are going to see all of the benefits of having a healthy vagus nerve, but there's even more.

1. Deep breathing is going to help to reduce stress and relieve anxiety.

2. It is going to help relieve pain. There are many techniques for deep breathing that focus completely on pain relief, and they work better as well as faster than any medication I have ever been given.

3. Deep breathing helps to improve a person's mood. It is actually a technique that is taught to children who have behavioral disorders as well as anger issues. Researchers understand that when we focus on our breathing and allow our bodies to stop that fight or flight

response, we are better able to control our own moods.

4. It helps to improve depression symptoms. One symptom that many people who have depression suffer from is a poor quality of sleep. However, when you practice deep breathing techniques, your quality of sleep is going to improve. It has also been found that deep breathing helps to reduce the heart rate of those that are struggling with depression as well as anxiety.

5. Deep breathing also helps to improve focus. Several studies have shown that by practicing deep breathing techniques for just 10 minutes, there was an immediate improvement of focus as well as a decrease in the person's blood pressure. Another study showed that by practicing deep breathing daily for just six weeks, test scores improved as well as rapid-fire test scores.

6. We spoke about OCD earlier in this book and how it is much more than just a desire to have a clean home. However, what we did not talk about is how hard OCD is to treat.

The good news is that deep breathing techniques can help with OCD symptoms. In fact, studies have shown that practicing deep breathing patients' symptoms improve drastically even to the point that they were able to reduce their medication dosages.

7. How many websites or eBooks have you seen lately that are focused on increasing one's energy? Maybe you have gone looking for a way to increase your energy. I have good news for you if you have any. Deep breathing exercises are going to help increase your energy levels. There is a very simple explanation for how this works. We already know that deep breathing helps to reduce stress, and it helps us to stay focused on the present. Because stress is reduced, the body has all of this energy that it was using by focusing on the stress, that is now freed up to be used for other things.

8. Deep breathing can actually help those that are suffering from obesity. Studies have shown that when a person uses deep breathing, they are able to overcome the

hunger pangs that they struggle with when they are trying to lose weight or when they are fasting. We should have known this because how many times do, and we see monks fasting without looking as if they are starving to death? Sure, their bodies may be hungry, but they are taking control away from their body instead of letting it control them. By practicing deep breathing techniques, a person may find that they are better able to stick to low-calorie diets or to fast without struggling with the hunger pangs that usually come with restricting food.

9. It helps with PTSD. There are so many people today that are suffering from PTSD for one reason or another. Some of our soldiers come home suffering from it, sometimes it is caused by a traumatic event that happened in childhood, but no matter what the reason deep breathing can help. When a person with PTSD practices deep breathing they are going to be able to sleep better, focus on what they are doing instead of getting distracted by the event that took place, they

are going to be able to take control of the anger that they feel, and they will be less irritable.

10. It can improve the quality of life of those that practice. There are so many benefits of practicing deep breathing that it is no wonder that research is showing that it can affect a person's entire life. What is even more amazing is that people often report feeling like they are finally experiencing life the way that it was meant to be experienced. They are able to focus on the tasks that they need to complete. Their productivity level increases dramatically. They are better able to get along with those around them. They begin focusing on their health, taking better care of themselves, and feeling better than ever before.

Is it really possible to change your life by doing something as simple as breathing? In short, yes. If you practice deep breathing techniques and you focus on doing them properly, you are going to see huge changes in your life. Remember, not only does deep breathing have its own benefits, but you are also going to see all of the benefits of stimulating your vagus nerve, which is what this is all about.

There are hundreds of different deep breathing techniques out there, many of them focusing on specific areas such as pain reduction or increasing energy. This means that you do not have to use the technique that I provided for you in this book. In fact, there are many guided, deep breathing techniques available for you to use online completely free. However, this was just an example for you so that you could see just how simple deep breathing is.

So come on, give it a shot. What do you have to lose? Deep breathing takes hardly any effort, and the benefits are so amazing.

Essential Motor Functions

Vagus Nerve Influence On The Oral Cavity

The **afferent** vagal nerve, which brings information to the brain and spinal cord, assesses the amount of food in the gastrointestinal tract, notably the stomach and intestines, and also determine the rate at which the food is processed; it also determines levels of stored fuel in circulation, and that is immediately available for energy. The vagus nerve transmits this information to the oral cavity, where it influences the desire—or lack of desire—for food intake.

Separately, the **efferent** vagal nerve, which sends information down from the brain to the gut region, assesses the rate at which the available nutrients are being absorbed, stored, or otherwise being utilized.

Another function of the "downward" efferent vagal nerve is to sense, within the gastrointestinal tract, the presence of two hormonal peptides, ghrelin and leptin, which are produced in the gut and known to affect appetite; either increasing or suppressing the urge to eat. The vagus nerve is believed to bring information about the levels of these hormones to the oral cavity, notably the taste buds on the tongue and elsewhere in the mouth.

The taste buds and other oral surfaces are not alone in detecting tastes; the gastrointestinal tract is also endowed with this capability, which explains why assessments of taste-detection in the gut further affect appetite, both positively and negatively.

Vagus Nerve Effects on Heartbeat

The heartbeat is stimulated and mediated by a series of nerve clusters in the myocardium, or heart muscle. Electrical impulses are sent via the vagus nerve to the sinoatrial node (also called the sinus node), at the top of the myocardium, directly above the right atrium. The impulses then travel downward through a series of nerve clusters: atrioventricular node, the bundle of His, right and left bundle branches, and finally, the Purkinje fibers. Each nerve cluster, in turn, contributes electrical impulses to simultaneously activate the right and left ventricles, causing the familiar heartbeat as blood enters the two atria, descends to the two ventricles, and is pumped out to either the aorta to reach the entire body or the pulmonary artery, for the trip back to the lungs for reoxygenation.

The vagus nerve intervenes in lowering the heart rate because the sinoatrial node, which is known as the heart's natural pacemaker, regulates the heartbeat. The right vagus nerve innervates (fills with nerve fibers) the sinoatrial node, and uses this connection to slow the heartbeat, which usually begins at a rate of up to 100 beats per second and needs to be slowed to 60 or 70 beats. Subsequent influences of the other nerve clusters may further lower the heartbeat.

A condition known as respiratory sinus arrhythmia (RSA) is a common, normal change that happens naturally during the cycle of breathing, as the heartbeat increases during inhalation and decreases during the exhale. This effect is mediated by vagal tone, which causes rising and falling of the diaphragm to open and close the lungs, but also varying pressure within the chest cavity that influences heart rate.

Vagus Nerve Control of Breathing

The vagus nerve is closely involved with the cycle of breathing, and for that reason, breathing exercises and other forms of managed breathing are credited by respected medical and physiological authorities with being able to affect vagal tone positively, and in turn, slow heart rate, ease tension, create a sense of calm.

The diaphragm is the largest (and strongest) muscle in our bodies. It is dome-shaped and located below the lungs and heart, positioned to separate the thoracic chest cavity (where the lungs are located) and the abdominal cavity. By creating an airtight seal between the two cavities, the diaphragm can affect the air pressure in the thoracic cavity. When the diaphragm contracts, it enlarges the volume of the thoracic cavity, causing a drop in air pressure. This causes the lungs to inflate, filling with air, this is an inhale. Conversely, when the diaphragm expands, the thoracic cavity's volume is reduced, increasing the air pressure and forcing the lungs to deflate, and exhale.

We breathe, automatically, unconsciously, every minute, every hour, every day. Each breath brings air into our lungs, air, which contains oxygen that is needed for our cells to function and survive. The air in the lungs fills millions of tiny air sacs, or alveoli, which are lined with capillaries carrying blood-enriched with hemoglobin; the hemoglobin contains iron atoms which bond easily with oxygen, which is then carried to every cell in our bodies.

Given the diaphragm's direct control over the cycle of breathing, it follows that conscious control of breathing may influence the diaphragm, reversing the cause and effect. Since the vagus nerve mediates the functions of the diaphragm, manipulation of the diaphragm is believed to influence the tonality of the vagus nerve.

Vagus Nerve Effects on The Digestive System

The vagus nerve plays a series of vital roles in the digestive system, helping to control the continuing process of food descending from the mouth, passing the epiglottis, entering the esophagus, passing the esophageal sphincter, entering the stomach where the vagus nerve ensures food is prepared for assimilation and pushed forward into the small intestine, where assimilation actually occurs. It further ensures the food continues to be digested as it continues on into the large intestine and the travers portion of the colon. Vagal fibers also extend into the liver and pancreas.

As it descends, the vagus nerve reaches and influences all components of the digestive system. Together these connections form the esophageal plexus. In this series of connections, the vagus nerve plays a diversity of roles in controlling the digestive process. One notable effect is the mediation of peristalsis, the automatic contractions, and expansions that move food from the stomach into the small intestine. When this process is malfunctioning, it can lead to a condition called gastroparesis, in which the contractions fail to move food through the stomach, causing loss of appetite, pain, nausea, and malnutrition.

The vagus nerve plays a critical health maintenance role in the gastroesophageal system by preventing acid reflux, which can lead to gastroesophageal reflux disease (GERD). It facilitates blocking gastric hydrochloric acid (HCL) from entering the esophagus by managing the pressure of the esophageal sphincter (which closes the opening at the top of the stomach).

CHAPTER 4
INFLAMMATION AND AUTOIMMUNE DISEASES

Nearly every autoimmune disease is caused by inflammation in the body. In fact, a great number of diseases, in general, are due to inflammation in the tissues. It is a big problem and one that pills can't really fix, though anti-inflammatories will lower it somewhat.

Inflammation has been linked to some of the deadliest diseases today, including diabetes, cancer, stroke, heart disease, and others. It has also been connected to autism and mental health issues, as well as a number of other brain diseases. Inflammation can kill you, but it's not entirely bad.

A study done by Dr. Harold A. Silverman at the Laboratory for Biomedical Science at the Feinstein Institute for Medical Research showed some interesting connections between inflammation and the vagus nerve. It showed that if the vagus nerve has a low tone, then the body is at higher risk for increased and chronic inflammation. This prolonged inflammation could cause issues like rheumatoid arthritis and other conditions associated with long term inflammation in the body.

What Is Inflammation?

Before we look further at how the vagus nerve influences inflammation, you should understand what inflammation is all about. It's an essential part of the immune system, so in small doses, it is actually something you want to happen in the body, to a certain point. Sometimes it seems to overload, and that's when it becomes too much to handle.

Inflammation is when the tissues swell and redden. They may become hot to the touch, as well. It is the natural immune response to something irritating. For example, if you get a splinter in your skin, it is viewed as a foreign object and an irritant. Your immune system responds by inflaming the idea to help the body expel and rid itself of the irritant.

However, irritants aren't just actual foreign bodies. They can be germs, bacteria, viruses, or even medications or treatments for other diseases, like chemicals, chemotherapy, or radiation. Specific areas of inflammation have names, usually ending in "itis" such as dermatitis, which is inflammation of the skin, or bronchitis, which is an inflammation of the bronchi.

Symptoms get worse as the inflammation gets worse. It will start out with heat, swelling, pain, and redness, moving on to loss of function of the area that is affected. An inflamed joint will become impossible to move, and inflamed bronchi will make it tough to breathe.

As the inflammation worsens, you will start to feel sick and tired. A fever may occur, as well, another sign that your immune system is working overtime to eliminate the disease that has invaded. Your body will pour all energy into fighting the bacteria or virus, and the fever raises your metabolism, making it possible for the body to produce more antibodies and white blood cells.

Blood vessels tend to dilate to allow more blood flow to the affected area, which is necessary to get the white blood cells to the area of inflammation. This also causes a lot of pain, which is another protective mechanism. You will tend not to move a body part that is hurting, and you'll keep it protected.

The swelling that becomes evident at the site of infection is due to more and more fluid and blood cells rushing to the area. Once the irritant has been dealt with, the fluid level drops, and the swelling goes down. You will notice this, particularly in the nose when you have a cold or flu. The extra fluid helps eliminate the viruses, but it makes it hard to breathe through your nose when it is all swollen inside, thanks to inflammation of the mucous membranes.

When there is an actual threat to the body, this immune system response is invaluable and could even save your life. Unfortunately, inflammation isn't always helpful, and if it occurs outside an actual threat, it can cause a lot of issues. In fact, it is the main reason we have an autoimmune disease, which is when the body's immune system mistakes its own cells for an intruder and fights against it.

While it started out as a part of a healthy, functioning body, inflammation has become rampant in our lives for a variety of reasons. The SAD (standard American diet) that so many enjoy triggers inflammation throughout the body. Things like sugar, processed grains, and food additives can all contribute to this. In addition, people use more medications than ever before. As I've mentioned, this was my personal trigger for vagus nerve damage, but it all starts with inflammation.

The problem here is that inflammation and chronic sickness create a terrible cycle. The illness creates inflammation, and the inflammation worsens the illness. Add in all the other factors in life that are contributing to the inflammation of everything, and you have a serious problem that is very difficult to fix.

How Much Inflammation is Too Much?

Since inflammation is obviously a very important part of the immune system, you don't want to eradicate it completely. When do you know that it's too much? That's the big question that everyone wants to know the answer to.

If you are sick, some inflammation is normal. For example, when your nasal membranes swell up as you have a cold, it's a normal part of fighting off the virus. This isn't overkilling, and it will help your body recover faster. The same goes for when you are injured. A scraped knee will tend to get red and swollen for a day or two, then it subsides. As long as your immune system is doing its job properly, you don't have to worry.

The problem starts when things get out of hand. If you're not sick or injured, but you are experiencing inflammatory responses, something may be wrong.

When multiple body parts become inflamed for apparently no reason, it can also be an indication that the immune system is malfunctioning. Where it may be normal for one knee to swell up due to an injury, even one you don't recall happening, it's not normal for your shoulders, knees, and wrists to swell, heat up, and get red. This would probably indicate an overload of inflammatory hormones.

Another indication that it may be too much inflammation is when it lasts longer than the average disease. Inflammatory symptoms that continue far beyond the usual 3-7 days for a virus or several days or weeks past what would be normal for an injury can indicate a poorly functioning immune system.

Your doctor can help you diagnose an inflammatory issue since it will also tend to show up in blood tests. However, your own experiences can also tell you if you have a problem. You know your body best and will be able to determine if there is something going on with it.

Autoimmune Diseases Caused by Inflammation

Once the body starts fighting its own cells, a war begins in you. This can be horribly uncomfortable, but it gets worse. When your immune system is busy fighting off an imaginary threat, it is more susceptible to other diseases sneaking in. You may find that if you suffer from an autoimmune disease, you also deal with a lot of colds and flu. You may feel like you catch every bug going by, and that's because you do. When the immune system is fighting this hard, it can't stop everything, and germs will get past the lowered protective barriers.

Autoimmune diseases are varied in how they present, but they all have one thing in common . . . the immune system is fighting against your own body. Here are some of the more common diseases associated with this issue.

Addison's disease: The adrenal glands are the affected organs in this disease. They produce several hormones, including androgen, aldosterone, and cortisol. Without these, the body can become quite imbalanced. You'll tend to lose weight, feel weak and exhausted, and your blood sugar will usually below. This also causes excess potassium to wind up in the blood, while sodium levels drop drastically.

Autoimmune vasculitis: When the immune system attacks blood vessels, it can cause serious issues. The resulting inflammation actually squeezes the arteries and veins, nearly closing them and preventing proper circulation. This causes some pretty obvious health risks that should be avoided.

Celiac disease: Also referred to as gluten sensitivity, this is actually an autoimmune disease where gluten causes the immune system to attack the small intestine when passing through. This results in inflammation and can cause leaky gut. It's a very serious disease, and even a small amount of gluten can trigger an immune response.

Grave's disease: This autoimmune disease causes the thyroid to overproduce hormones. Too many thyroid hormones will speed up your metabolism and can speed up your heart rate, cause extreme weight loss, anxiety, and heat intolerance. One of the most notable and unpleasant symptoms of Grave's disease is eyes that bulge out of the head.

Hashimoto's: You may have heard of this disease, which also affects the thyroid. However, unlike Grave's, Hashimoto's causes the thyroid to stop functioning properly, and it has the opposite effect on the body, causing weight gain. You'll tend to be sensitive to cold, and your hair will fall out. It can also cause goiters, or the swelling of the thyroid to the point that it forms a large lump on the neck.

Inflammatory bowel disease: Commonly known as IBD, there are a few sub-diseases under this. It refers to inflammation of the intestinal walls, but depending on where it is, the disease has a specific name.

Crohn's disease affects any part of the digestive tract, even outside the intestines. It can cause inflammation from anus to mouth, though it generally only affects a certain section of the GI tract.

Ulcerative colitis is specifically limited to the colon and rectum and is caused by massive inflammation there.

Lupus: Systemic lupus erythematosus is another autoimmune disease that you have probably heard of. Originally thought to be a skin issue, it has now become evident that lupus affects many internal organs as well. Most commonly, the immune system attacks the brain, kidneys, joints, and the heart, causing pain and fatigue.

Multiple sclerosis: MS is one of the more deadly autoimmune diseases. In this case, the nervous system is attacked, and the protective myelin around the nerves is destroyed. This results in poor communication between the body and brain, which makes people feel numb and gradually lose the ability to walk and balance. It slowly robs the affected person of their ability to move and do things on their own, even affecting speech, until eventually, it affects even heart and lung function.

Psoriasis: Everyone grows new skin cells on a regular basis, and we are constantly losing or shedding old skin cells. With psoriasis, the immune system attacks the skin and causes the cells to grow far too fast. They build up in patches and become inflamed and itchy. Psoriasis can also pass to the joints and cause a form of arthritis that is very painful.

Rheumatoid arthritis: This form of autoimmune disease involves the joints. Your immune system goes after the joints, and you'll find that your joints tend to be hot, red, and stiff. It can be so painful as to affect your daily activities.

Sjögren's syndrome: In this particular syndrome, the glands that keep your mouth and eyes lubricated are affected. It can also attack the joints, causing inflammation there, but the most common symptoms are dry eyes and mouth.

Type 1 diabetes mellitus: Your pancreas is responsible for secreting insulin to regulate the blood sugar levels throughout the body. However, with this type of diabetes, your immune system actually fights against the pancreas. This destroys the cells that are responsible for making insulin and causes the patient to take insulin via injection for life.

These are just a few of the many autoimmune diseases that can affect you. They tend not to be constant but can have what is referred to as flares, where the symptoms become much worse for a period of time. This often coincides with high stress, sickness, or other issues that place more pressure on the body.

Signs that you have an inflammation problem or an autoimmune disease include:

-Aches and pains

-Swelling

-Redness in specific areas

-Low-grade fever

-Fatigue

-Hair falling out

-Rashes on skin

-Tingling in the extremities

-Difficulty focusing

-Memory issues

If these symptoms persist, even after you should be over a regular cold or other illness, it's possible your immune system is attacking your body itself. The resulting inflammation could become worse and then improve, but it will likely continue to be an issue until the underlying problem is resolved.

While immune system responses that cause disease are becoming more common now, it may be brought under control by using vagus nerve stimulation, which actually reduces inflammation.

Managing Inflammation with Vagus Nerve Stimulation

Inflammation is controlled by the vagus nerve, and when it is low in tone, you will find that there is a lot more inflammation in your body. When the nerve is stimulated, it lets the immune system know that it should calm down. The result is less chronic inflammation and better health.

Your immune system can malfunction just like everything else in the body, but when it does, it has widespread effects. Chronic inflammation will cause poor health and can even result in death if it gets bad enough. That's right, and your own body can actually kill you if the inflammation gets out of control. This is why people die from autoimmune diseases.

It's obviously best to prevent mistaken immune system responses, but the current method is to dose people up with medications that lower the immune system. These are the same drugs used to treat cancer, and they have their own side effects. It's also not a good idea to restrict your immune system for long periods of time, as this can leave you open to a lot of other diseases and will limit your lifestyle.

It's far better to aim for natural methods of reducing inflammation. Eating a healthy diet and eliminating sugar and processed foods from your diet is a good start, but frequent stimulation of the vagus nerve is also useful. It will help your body lower the inflammation and prevent the creation of more white blood cells, which can be an issue when there are too many of them.

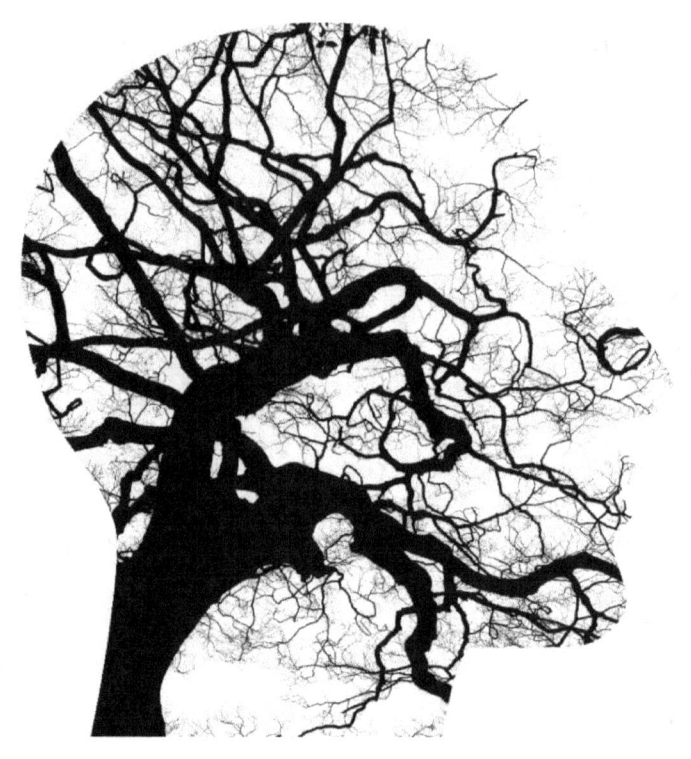

CHAPTER 5
VAGUS NERVE MALFUNCTIONS

In the vegetative nervous system, the misalignment of the atlas can compress the nerve bundles and adversely affect its function.

Similarly, if you tighten the antenna cable with a clamp, you cannot watch TV programs. Similarly, electrical impulses passing through the nervous system can be disrupted and weakened or lost.

What do you think will happen next to an organ connected to that system?

The vagus nerve is particularly affected by atlas shifts. This nerve compression can cause so-called vagal symptoms.

The vagus nerve system can be altered mainly in three ways:

- **Communication of an organ with the brain (through glutamate),**
- **Communication within the brain (from NTS or DMV)**
- **Communication from the brain to other**

areas of the body, such as the heart, liver, and intestine.

Diseases of Vagus Nerve

The loss or alteration of the function of the vagus nerve, for example, in case of cervical arthrosis, will result in a loss of parasympathetic innervation for a very large number of structures with great consequences for the vital functions of the individual.

The main effects of vagus nerve damage can include an increase in blood pressure and heart rate. On the other hand, vagal hyperstimulation can induce severe bradycardia, the onset / worsening of an atrioventricular block, and even the death of the patient.

This, for example, occurs in cases of asphyxia during erotic practices or even with shirt neck collars or too tight ties

Symptoms and signs of vagus compromise may include:

- Nausea;
- He retched;
- Constipation;

- Diarrhea;
- Anxiety;
- Tremors;
- Dysphagia (difficulty swallowing);
- Difficulty moving the mouth;
- Stomach acid;
- Dizziness;
- Dizziness;
- Face blush;
- Tachycardia or bradycardia (depending on the type of vagal alteration);
- Hypotension or arterial hypertension;
- Pain and stiffness in the neck;
- Headache
- Pallor;
- Cold sweats;
- Reduced salivation;
- Difficult digestion;
- Cerebral hypoperfusion;
- Fainting;

- Collapse.

DIAGNOSIS OF THE VAGUS NERVE

Many symptoms of vagal inflammation are nonspecific and can make diagnosis difficult and delayed.

For example, gastrointestinal symptoms such as gastric acid, vomiting, and constipation can mistakenly direct a doctor to be possible gastrointestinal and non-neurological causes. Heart disease symptoms may also indicate heart problems purely.

Doctors suspect inflammation of the vagus nerve only with a very accurate medical history (patient data collection, symptoms, habits, family pathology ...) related to physical examination including the head, neck, chest, and abdomen.

In many cases, differential diagnosis is only useful by instrumental examinations such as ultrasound scans, CT scans, and/or magnetic resonance imaging associated with common laboratory tests.

Diagnosis may require the advice of a neurologist, orthopedic surgeon, cardiologist, or even a psychiatrist. For severe heart conditions, a series of diagnostic tools may be required, including:

- An objective examination of the heart.
- Blood pressure measurement.
- ECG (ECG);
- Chest radiograph.
- Heart enzymes.
- Coronary angiography with potential angioplasty (coronary angiography).
- Cardiac ultrasound (Echo Color Doppler);
- Echocardiogram by the transesophageal route.
- Stress echocardiogram (eco-stress);
- 24-hour halter.

An electroencephalogram is also helpful in cases of severe neurological symptoms.

TREATMENT

There is no single treatment to resolve vagal inflammation. The specific treatment is based on the underlying causes of the inflammation. In some cases, patients can benefit from applying medical methods such as Valsalva or carotid massage.

Valsalva law consists of forced exhalation with the

closed glottis. A carotid massage consists of pressing two or three fingers in the neck area corresponding to the carotid sinus. Vagus nerve stimulation is sometimes used as a tool to reduce anxiety and psychosomatic stress

How to activate the vagus nerve to regenerate the body

Exercise to stimulate the vagus nerve

A very simple technique that you can perform anywhere is to make a conscious breath. This is the only function of the autonomic nervous system that can be regulated and promotes relaxation, elimination of toxins, concentration, and calm.

To perform abdominal or diaphragmatic breathing, you should only:

- Inspire through the nose slowly, mentally counting to 4.
- Hold the air in the lungs, counting to 6, and contracting the abdomen.
- Exhale counting to 4, slightly contracting the lips.

Try to do this several times every day and,

especially in a stressful situation. Do it slowly and deeply, becoming aware of air travel throughout the body.

In addition to contributing to relaxation, this exercise, in the long term, can help lower blood pressure, improve heart rate, improve immune function, and reduce anxiety.

Other tips to stimulate the vagus nerve

- Place a damp and fresh cloth on the face.
- Drink a glass of cold water quickly.
- Lie on an inclined surface, head down.
- Eat a diet that contains vegetables, nuts, and fruits, avoiding excess cereals (especially refined ones), oxidized vegetable oils, sugars, dairy products, and processed food.
- Keep in mind that your body has a great capacity for healing. Learn to work with him, and increase your ability to register to understand what may be happening to you and know when to turn in search of a professional who can help you.

Abdominal toning exercises are excellent for this purpose, clarifying that the abdominals are not only the repetitive lifting of the torso or legs, but there are other alternatives with which to work in this area of the body. Some abs are:

- Upper abs: the classics, up and down the torso.
- Lower abs: raising the legs to 90º (or whatever you can) and lowering them.
- Crunches: Perform at the same time upper abs and knees approach to the chest.
- Bring legs to the chest and embrace them inhaling, then stretch them and suspend them briefly at 30º concerning the ground.
- Plates: Lean on the elbows to the width of the arms and hands together. Stretched body and back, you rest on the toes — 30 seconds to 1 minute.
- Platform posture: You hold on your hands and with arms stretched to shoulder width, keep the body aligned from neck to

toe for about 30 seconds to 1 minute for greater difficulty do not rest on the toes of the back, but the insteps.

- Legs in suspension 30º: with the pointed feet and the torso and hands resting on the ground. Take a deep breath or pump until you can't stand it anymore and lower your legs. Try to endure more and more time.

Constant abdominal strengthening is necessary for you to tone the abdominal wall so that your organs have enough space to operate properly.

Exercises, where the abdomen is stretched, are important - and not only contractions - as in the case of the last 3, because with them, we undo possible accumulated tensions in these muscles that hinder the proper functioning of the vagus nerve.

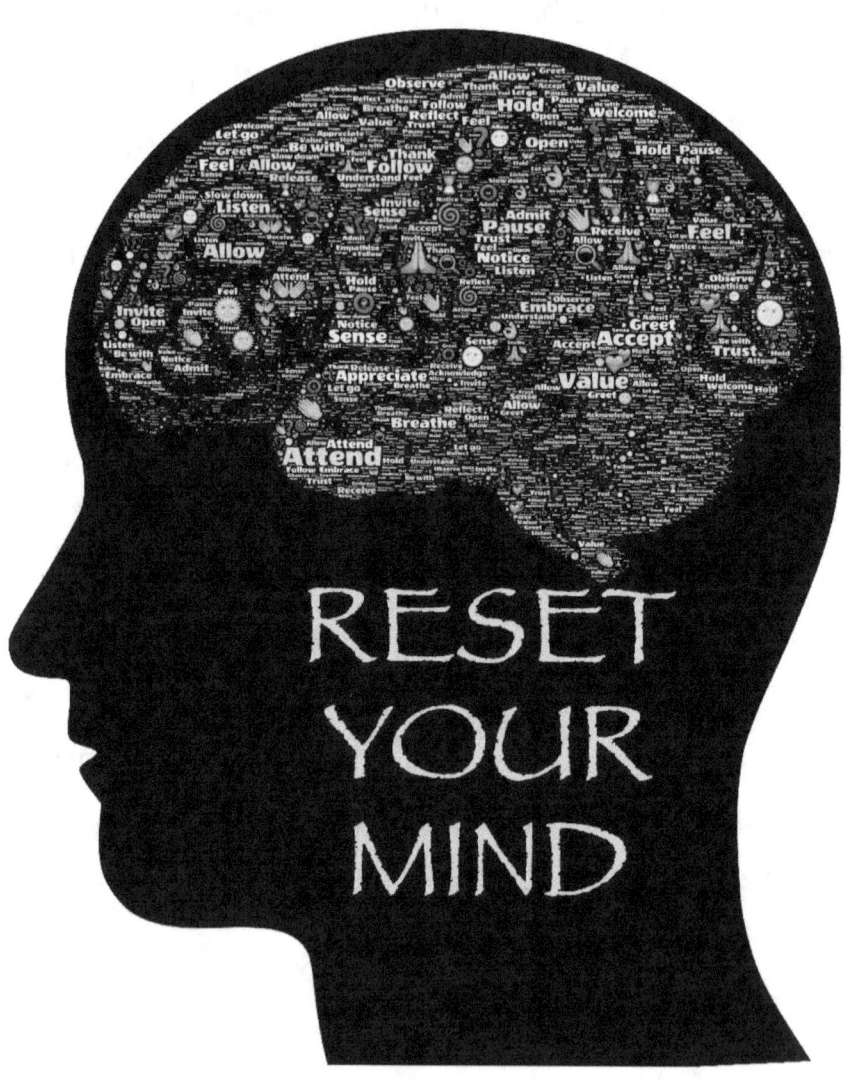

CHAPTER 6
POLYVAGAL WORLD

Did you know that play has a definition? According to play expert, Dr. Peter Gray, in order to qualify as truly play, it must have these five characteristics:

- An activity that is chosen on your own and directed on your own
- Engaged in for the sake of the activity and not for some reward
- Includes some sort of structure or set of rules
- Employs an imaginary element of some kind
- Be done in an alert, conscious frame of mind

Based on those criteria, much of what we do these days is not truly considered play.

For many years, children were allowed to play on their own, but now we have changed all that. Children spend most of their time either in school, doing homework, or in some sort of extracurricular activity that the parents have deemed important. I remember as a child, I used to walk outside and encounter other children playing all the time, but now children go outside to be met with silent streets. No one has time to go outside and play in their yards because they are too busy being shuttled to ballet, art class, piano lessons, after-school activities, organized sports, something. Always something else. While these activities alone would not be a problem, it is the fact that they have now so completely taken over children's lives to the detriment of free time.

Parents feel the need to supervise every moment of their child's day, not only to watch them constantly but also to direct them in all of those activities. There are seemingly no independent moments for children anymore, and certainly, nothing that involves risk. I have seen parents upset at their child for climbing a tree, when, in fact, tree climbing is a time-honored activity that ought to be enjoyed by every child. We have lost the notion of free play.

How does this relate to the polyvagal theory, you might ask? Well, by structuring our children's day to the last minute, every day, we have set up a framework for them to grow up in. Their neural development is still happening during these years, and they are now only experiencing a rigid structure, rules placed on them by someone else, a play directed not by themselves but by some outward force. And all activities in a completely safe environment, no risks involved anywhere.

You may ask why any of that might bear on the neurological development. As the polyvagal theory teaches, if we can train our vagus pathways to respond more appropriately to situations that have caused us anxiety in the past, then it stands to reason that we can train our neurological pathways only to feel safe in a structured environment. By not allowing our children to have adequate time to play freely, we have trained them that they are only safe in structured moments. Imagine then, when the child turns into an adult, and no one is telling them every step to take, every rule they must follow. Many of us do not need to imagine it now, because it is exactly what we felt when we became that adult ourselves.

I mentioned risk for a reason as well. Growing up in an environment where you are never in any sort of self-directed risky situation means you will never learn that you have the capacity to survive these minor risks. Here I am not talking about purposely living in a constant state of fear or actual danger, but rather just allowing your child to do things that involve minor risk. Climbing a tree comes to mind. Wrestling with other kids, riding a bike, swinging from a tree swing. These things prove to the child that they can handle minor fear that they can survive a certain amount of risk, and they can take charge of their own environment.

These are vital lessons to learn as children, and the lack of these lessons carries on into adulthood. A child who does not know how to problem solve in freestyle play will be an adult who does not know how to problem solve on the job.

Perhaps this lack of play as children has also contributed to the rise in anxiety in adults in recent years. Imagine entering adulthood, feeling completely unprepared, and having no idea how to prepare oneself. Not even knowing what you lack in so you can go out and teach it to yourself. We have all this technology at our fingertips, yet the only thing we really need to do is use our imaginations in free playtime.

I read of one community that may have found a solution to this issue. They have a community playtime during which families bring their children specifically for unstructured playtime. The only structure allowed is the meeting time and the agreed-upon playground, and an adult or two to provide light supervision in case of real emergencies and to prevent truly life-threatening risky behavior. Otherwise, children from kindergarten through fifth grade are allowed to freely roam, playing whatever games they choose, and interacting with whomever they wish in that environment.

Free play is an integral part of the story we tell ourselves as adults. It has an impact on what we perceive about our own abilities and the dangers existing in our surroundings. The free play tells us what we are truly capable of and forces us to stretch our minds and bodies to overcome obstacles and solve problems.

Let's bring free playback into our world.

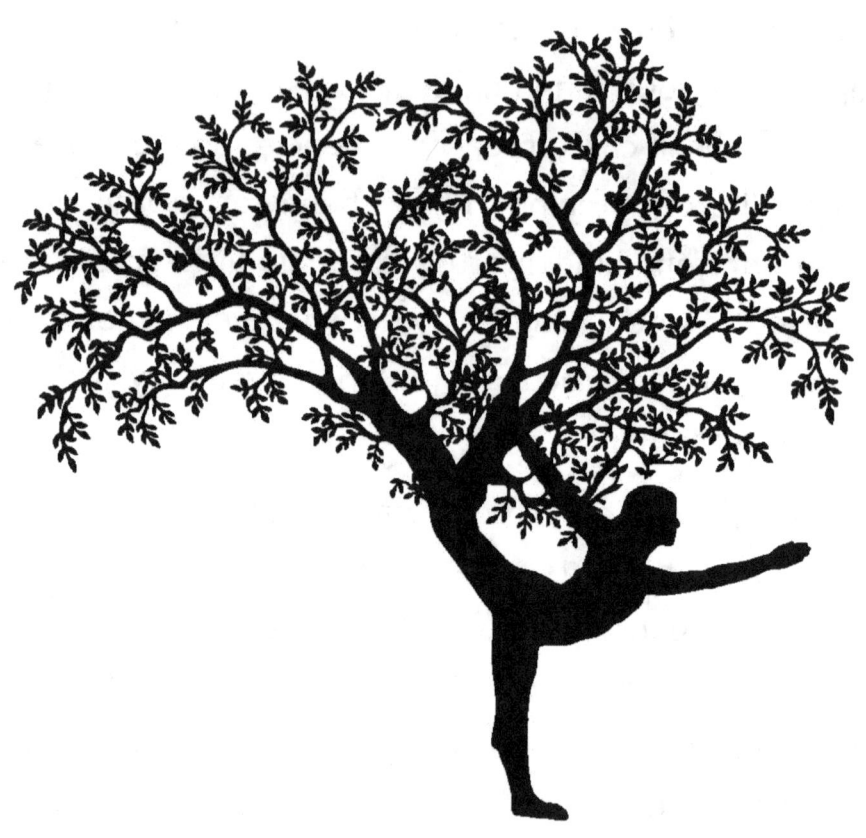

CHAPTER 7
POLYVAGAL AND AUTISM

Autism Spectrum Disorder

Autism is a large and complex disorder that spans an entire spectrum, to the point that one definition for autism cannot really be summed up in totality in just one sentence. However, generally speaking, autism is a sensory disorder, affecting different individuals to different degrees and manifesting in different ways for each individual.

In the United States alone, one in fifty-nine children are autistic, with one in thirty-seven boys and one in one hundred-fifty-one girl, and the numbers of diagnoses seem to be going up. Whether this is due to a rising incidence of the condition or rising awareness is not yet completely known. Most of these children are not diagnosed until after the age of four, although there have been cases of children as young as two years old being diagnosed.

Being a spectrum disorder means there is a range

of symptoms affecting social and communication skills, as well as motor and language skills, to some degree – sometimes greater, sometimes less.

Often the autistic individual sees social cues as danger signs rather than invitations to engage, or they could completely lack those social instincts needed to navigate in a social world. They may see a hug as an attack, a smile as a grimace, or an exuberant greeting as a grating intrusion on their sense of peace.

In recent years though, there has been some progress made on figuring out what may be the cause of or contributing factors to autism.

One thing that is said now to be a factor is inflammation and immune problems – specifically neuro-inflammation and neuro-immune abnormalities. If the vagus nerve helps to reduce inflammation, perhaps some people with autism will be receiving help in a short while, but that is the neurological, biological part of the struggle with autism. We are going to focus now on the connection between the mind and the body and how it relates to the world of the autistic person.

Mind-body Connection

However, one thing that is becoming more apparent is that a method of therapy called mind-body connectedness is showing promise in the autistic world.

On a daily deep level, those with autism contend with a problem connecting their mind to their body and letting it stay there. The noise that surrounds them is overwhelming, causing their senses to overload. The only relief they have is through withdrawal. Perhaps we can offer some relief in some other way.

Those on the spectrum have a problem recognizing the way their body feels in a safe state. Rather than an inability to recognize safety physically, though that is also often present, this is the inability to understand that their state of mind is safe. It does not seem safe to them, so they need added reinforcement to recognize that state and allow their bodies to stay in it. Think of it this way – if you are born within a state of fight or flight, your body will come to recognize that as what is your normal. Anything outside that normal becomes a sign of danger. Bring that body to a quiet, calm state, and those neurons will fire off warnings and danger signals, thinking there is some sort of danger to be fought off.

One thing to remember, first, is that the goal for anyone on the autism spectrum is not to become *normal*, or the same as most people around them. They are normal already, just their normal. Their senses become overwhelmed, but this does not indicate that their senses are wrong. The person with autism has heightened sensitivity, but that also translates into heightened perception, heightened appreciation for beauty or music, a heightened ability to see or hear things that slip past other people.

Our society is not "autism-friendly." Our society is not built in a way that is sensitive to those with sensory disabilities. There is always some noise or flashing lights, weird smells, bright colors, fast-moving crowds, or traffic, and then we place the autistic person in numerous social settings that are dependent on only instincts. They are left in a crowd wondering where the social engagement manual was hidden because they didn't get to read it. They are placed in schools where other kids seem to know exactly how to act instinctively, while they are left alone to struggle through mistake after mistake. They are placed in social settings where they can see a hierarchy exists, but they have no idea how to function within that hierarchy. This would be absolutely terrifying, and it is no wonder they often shut down.

Even with all this, there is no reason to bring them to a state that looks like everyone else. What they most need is to be brought into a state where they are more comfortable, a place where they can be safe and happy in their own body, whatever that state looks like. The individual with autism will have his or her own happy optimal state, and that is what the caregiver or therapist or loved one should focus on helping them find.

Polyvagal theory approaches autism from a different direction than many other treatments and therapy models. It looks at the person's neurological state and assumes that something has caused this person's biology to immobilize them, perhaps from birth. Immobilization is a very real, very biological thing. We know that this state exists now. It is further than just freezing, or even dissociation. It is immobilization where a person literally cannot move.

They cannot access their body in a functional state, and it is happening to them on a neurological level. The autistic person may have something happening to his body that he cannot control. Instead, it has been taken over by the sympathetic nervous system.

This is why therapy from a polyvagal viewpoint will approach the body of the person on the spectrum first. The belief is that the autistic person is so disconnected from their body that they cannot control it sometimes. They cannot control the slide into a meltdown, and they do not know how to keep themselves in that safe space. There is also much evidence that says they do not recognize a safe space when it does happen. Even a state of stillness can be seen as a threat to the autistic person. Perhaps they have only ever experienced stillness as a response to perceived danger, their body having always interpreted the stimuli around them as signals of danger. They need to be taught that stillness can happen in safety as well.

Researchers used to believe that the brain reaches a certain point and never changes after that, but more recent studies have called that conclusion into question. Now the science of neuroplasticity is giving us indications that the brain can change and grow, even into adulthood.

How does this impact autism? This thought impacts autism in that we now believe the autistic brain can change, be taught to tolerate sensory stimuli, at least to a better degree than they are used to. This can lead to more comfort for the person living with autism, as well as provide more weapons for their arsenal in combatting difficult, complex social issues. While we do not want to change who they are, we do wish to give them some relief from their isolation. They may feel betrayed by their body. They can learn that they do not have to feel betrayed anymore, but instead can come into unity with their body, and bring it to a place of safety.

There are some therapies that focus on this specifically. Some chiropractors have also seen improvement when working with autistic children.

The point of this sort of therapy is to get yourself into a safe and open position and learn that there is no danger there. For the sake of your loved one with autism, you are tasked with creating that safety for them when they are doing an exercise like this.

Allow them to have space, trust that they can

improve, trust that they have the ability to think things through on their own. Let them have that moment to climb up the vagal ladder on their own, while you create a safe space around them for them to accomplish this goal.

When working with an autistic child, the activities to enhance the brain-body connection can be simple.

I have seen a teacher cut out dinosaur shapes for a child who loved dinosaurs to use in learning his place values for math. She made different sizes, then baby dinosaurs, and lined them up to each represent different place values. This is a form of brain-body connection because the child could manipulate the dinosaurs and connect that physical touch with a learned fact. He was connecting his body to his mind.

Mind-body therapies include things like meditation, prayer, guided imagery, biofeedback, yoga, and cognitive behavioral therapy.

CHAPTER 8
VAGUS NERVE AND ANXIETY DISORDER

Anxiety Disorder has been misunderstood. First, it is produced from the body. Preconditions are first set by the body, and then the mind can enforce it. Of course, a trained mind can make it easier to cope with an anxiety disorder as it is an out of balance state. The body cannot find the equilibrium between the relaxation and stress modes.

The anxiety caused by the mind will go itself for a month because the body and mind will get used to the new psychological fears, and a healthy body will find a way to go to the relaxation mode. I would emphasize a healthy or well-functioning body because only when the body is healthy will it find the way. It is designed to go into relaxation mode. No help is needed. And body-induced anxiety will keep longer, maybe years. The easiest way to treat it is to treat the body.

The vagus nerve is going to be the tenth of twelve pairs of cranial nerves and, in addition, will be the longest to the entire body. In truth, the word vagus indicates "vagabond" in Latin, together with beautifully illustrates the highway of the nerve extending through several organs of the body. The vagus nerve is produced to the cranial box, exactly in the spinal cord, as well as additionally will go into the neck construction on two limbs as well as getting the abdomen passing out of the various organs across the book.

The vagus nerve intervenes in the understanding of the respiratory mucous membranes as well as directs the rhythm, strength, and frequency of breathing. It negatively impacts the pharynx, the larynx, the esophagus, the trachea, and the bronchi and also administering nerve fibers to the heart, stomach, pancreas, and liver. Although additionally, it functions the inverse mission; that is, it gets signals coming from the internal organs as well as directs them together with the mind to be digested. While most likely probably the most intriguing thing is definitely the relationship between the vagus nerve in addition to anxiety as additionally, it sends signals of nervousness or calm, anger, or relaxation. To understand the website link between the vagus nerve in addition to the anxiety, we've to master the main nervous system consists of two "opposite" techniques that constantly send information on the human mind.

The sympathetic nervous system prepares us for action, and consequently, it mainly feeds stress hormones like adrenaline and cortisol. The parasympathetic nervous system intervenes in rest and relaxation. In practice, both strategies work as accelerators and decelerators. The sympathetic nervous system boosts as well as influences us as the parasympathetic nervous system can help us relax and reduce the pace; consequently, it will make use of neurotransmitters for instance acetylcholine, which cuts down on the heart rate in addition to blood pressure level to make sure that the organs work slower. The characteristics of the vagus nerve adjust the parasympathetic system. It intervenes in features that are numerous, from mouth motions to heartbeat, and, when impacted, it's in a position to lead to various signs. A number of the vagus nerve works in our body are: - It is able to assist control heartbeat, regulates muscle mass motions and also will keep the pace of breathing.- It maintains the functionality of the intestinal tract, making it easy for the contraction of the belly in addition to intestine muscles to process foods.- Facilitates relaxation after a tense situation or even suggests we are in danger and we do not have to bring down the guard.- Send sensory information on the mind about organ quality.

When we are put through difficult conditions, the sympathetic nervous system is activated. If the pressure persists and we cannot switch off the biological effect which activates it, it won't pass the time, which is a great deal of before problems appear. With brain amount, that needs the activation of two pathways: the hypothalamus-pituitary-adrenal axis along with the mind intestine axis. The brain does react to anxiety as well as strain by increasing the development of hormones (CRFs) that travel from the hypothalamus on the pituitary gland where they result in the release of some other hormone (ACTH), that trips with the bloodstream on the adrenal glands to market cortisol in addition to adrenaline induction, which function as body 's body's immune system suppressors in addition to inflammatory precursors, and that is exactly why when we really feel anxious and pressured we're ill also and readily, in conclusion, we're competent to end up experiencing depression, an ailment that's attached to an inflammatory brain impact. And that way was not enough, persistent stress and anxiety result in heightened glutamate in the human mind, a neurotransmitter that, when produced in additional, depression, causes anxiety, and migraine. Furthermore, a great deal of cortisol cuts down on the quantity of the hippocampus, the element of the human mind to blame for the improvement of new memories. The involvement of the vagus nerve will result in issues as dizziness, gastrointestinal problems, arrhythmias, difficulty in breathing, and the disproportionate emotional responses. In truth, as the vagus nerve can't cause the leisure signal, the sympathetic nervous system is going to keep prosperous, and that will result in the person to respond also and impulsively are impacted by anxiety. It is also curious that analysis produced at the Faculty of Miami found the general vagal tone is transmitted from mom to child. Women experiencing anxiety, depression, or perhaps having a lot of anger during pregnancy had a reduced vagal exercise, and also, the kids of theirs likewise showed substandard vagal activity and reduced quantities of dopamine and serotonin. Three vagal stimulation techniques: the way you are able to cope with the vagus nerve? The general vagal tone is an inner purely natural method, and that should be on the exercise of the vagus nerve. The improved vagal tone sparks the parasympathetic nervous system, meaning we're competent to relax quicker after a tense circumstance, and also, this may have a great impact on the psychological harmony of ours and on health on the entire.

Many say that the anxiety disorder-caused symptoms are the effect of the anxiety itself. Mind-triggered anxiety is the cause, and body symptoms are affected. But, it is not so with a body-triggered anxiety disorder. It is both the anxiety and body symptoms that are caused by the body not being able to find equilibrium. Anxiety and body symptoms are both effects of something else, which is the cause.

For instance, a simple example is a small hiatal hernia (stomach), which irritates the vagus nerve in the hiatus. Thus, the body is the cause, and the mind follows. The other way is also true that psychological stresses will bring physiological symptoms. But it will not go for long. It will be stabilized soon.

The nervous system that maintains the balance between anxiety (fight or flight) and relaxation can be considered as a loop. Most of the organs are connected to this loop and are guided to operate into two modes: 1) fight or flight and 2) relaxation.

This loop is comprised of the vagus nerve and the nerves coming from the spinal cord. The vagus nerve itself is comprised of two branches: the dorsal branch and the ventral one (polyvagal theory).

Mind-driven anxiety is a broken balance in mind due to psychological causes. And Body-induced anxiety is a broken balance in the periphery (spinal and vagus nerves). The nerves can be disturbed in their path. They can be pinched. The vagus nerve travels along the path, which begins from the medulla located in the brainstem to all the organs. It is the longest cranial nerve. Thus, it is logical that some muscular-skeletal pressure can affect the vagus nerve along its path. Based on experiences of osteopaths, physiotherapists the most vulnerable places where the mechanical pressure can happen to the vagus nerve are two: 1) atlas-axis joint and 2) hiatus in the diaphragm (hiatal hernia).

Atlas is the upper cervical vertebrae, also known as C1. The misalignment of the atlas can put pressure on the vagus nerve that is located there. When the suboccipital muscles are stiff or tense, the atlas-axis joint can't function properly. A well-qualified osteopath or chiropractor may address the misalignment of the atlas.

And as mentioned, the vagus nerve irritation also can come from a hiatal hernia. In this case, the stomach puts pressure on the vagus while it goes through hiatus. A well-qualified osteopath or chiropractor may address the hiatal hernia.

The symptoms of a compressed or pinched vagus nerve are too many and manifest differently in different persons. The most common symptoms are anxiety, nausea, heartburn, tachycardia, vertigo, headache, sense of the lump in the throat, cold hands and cold feet, diarrhea, constipation, sweating, and many others.

The vagus nerve can be compressed or irritated at the diaphragm area. The diaphragm can be tensed or become tender. Abnormal breathing or slouched position may contribute to the creation of trigger points in the diaphragm. Trigger point therapy or osteopathic diaphragm release may help to release the tension and eliminate the trigger points located in the diaphragm.

First, observe if your anxiety depends on your postural changes of the body. Notice how your anxiety behaves when you are sitting or standing up when slouched. Try to notice if your neck position change can increase anxiety. Most of the anxiety disorder cases are due to mechanical causes which may compress or pinch some certain nerves. Nerves play an important role in blood supply by dilating the blood capillaries.

It is important to stress that many people have bodily symptoms without anxiety. In such a case, the vagus nerve is not involved in these symptoms. Only when the anxiety follows the bodily symptoms, the chances are high that the vagus nerves are involved directly in the scenario where the vagus is responsible for all. It would be normal to have mind-induced anxiety directly following some new symptoms but not continuously all year. The person will get used to symptoms after some time. Thus if the anxiety goes repeatedly and continuously following the bodily symptoms, then it is body-induced anxiety where the vagus nerve is involved.

The first step to help the body recover is to do some gentle exercises. It is better to begin for the first three months with the *Ping Shuai gong* three two-times a day than to combine with or switch to the *Zhan Zhuang* exercise. *Zhan Zhuang* is a big secret.

Biking is also a very helpful exercise for anxiety but should be associated with an internal qigong exercise. External exercises are good to burn stress, but after doing them, they leave us exhausted, while internal exercise, on the contrary, leaves us refreshed and energized.

We wanted to say that if you know that the cause of the symptoms is the neck, then you have to treat the neck. If the problem is located in the abdomen, then you have to focus on the abdominal massage to treat the abdominal trigger points. But when you don't know the cause, then it is better to exercise the *Zhan Zhuang*. Moreover, it is typical of the anxiety disorder, and then usually, the symptoms are located elsewhere different from the cause. The pain is here in a part of the body, but the cause of the pain is far away. The symptoms of anxiety disorder are tricky by misleading the sufferer and the doctor.

The *Zhan Zhuang* will enable the body to build new neural pathways by giving the body new ways of communication of information through the electromagnetic medium. Start the exercise for as few as 15 seconds in the beginning as you are not used to it. And then gradually increase the time to 15 minutes at least. Fifteen minutes is the minimum for seeing noticeable improvements. Twenty minutes is better. The healing process starts with 15 minutes, and the max time to practice is 40 minutes. Keep in mind not to exert the body too much. It is important that the upper body remains relaxed.

Whenever you experience new symptoms, it means that your body is experimenting with new neural pathways for achieving the equilibrium. So, the setbacks and the new symptoms are indications of healing. The healing process is not a linear process. It goes forth and back. Further, the healing effect is accumulative, which means, in the beginning, the results seem zero, but after some time, the healing appears instantly.

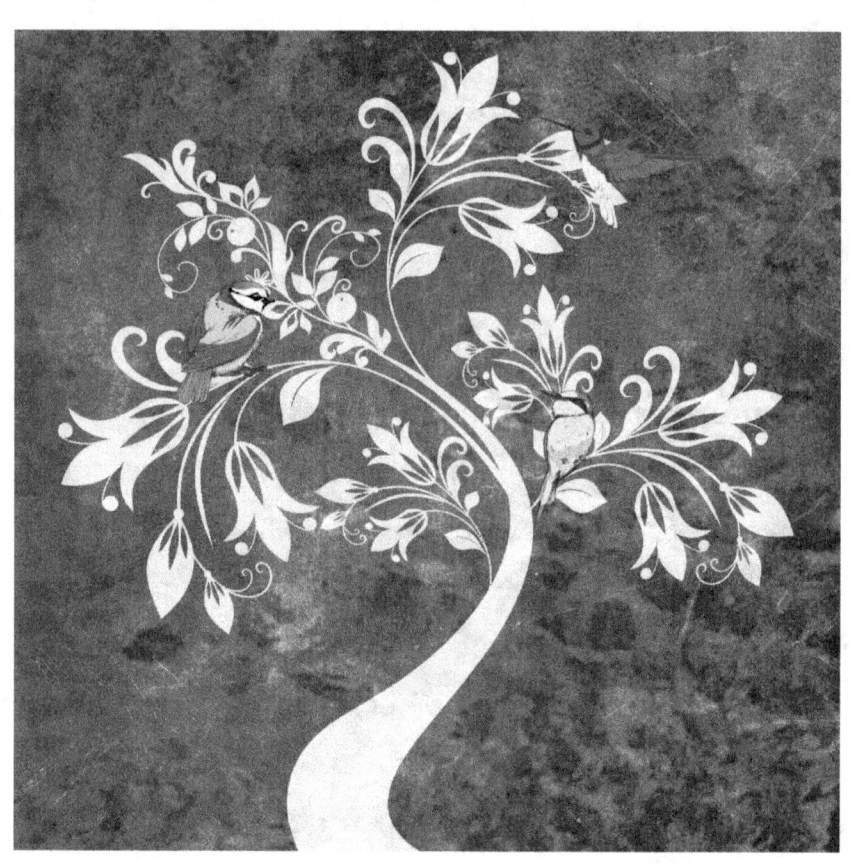

CHAPTER 9

UNDERSTANDING ANXIETY, PTSD, TRAUMA, AND DEPRESSION

What is Stress

Stress is a word that is often heard and talked about but truly, not fully understood. Some people consider stress as an event that happens in their lives, like losing a job or experiencing an accident or injury. Some people, on the other hand, would say that stress is the behavior of the body towards certain events such as nail-biting or anxiety.

In actuality, stress involves both the event and response of the body and mind to the so-called stressor (source of stress). When a person undergoes a situation, it is automatically evaluated by the mind mentally. The mind decides if the situation is a threat, then generates logic on how to deal with the situation at hand, and if the person has the skill to solve the problem. If it is decided that the skills acquired by the person are not enough to handle the problem, then the situation is labeled "stressful." If the situation is something the person can handle, then it is considered otherwise.

There are many sources of stress. Contrary to common belief, it is not always sourced from a negative situation. It could also be caused by positive situations like a job promotion or a new baby. The body experiences stress even in these positive changes because it has to adapt to new challenges. For some people, being flooded with added work and activities could cause enormous stress. Another good example of a positive situation that can cause stress is pregnancy or giving birth. For a mother, especially that is experiencing pregnancy for the first time, the body experiences enormous change. These changes may cause imbalances on the body, therefore releasing stress hormones. When the baby is born, both the father and mother will experience changes in their lifestyle, and if not properly conditioned for these changes, the situation also triggers stress.

Even if you don't struggle with anxiety and panic attacks on a daily basis, internalized stress can still silently wreak havoc on your body and mind, leaving you incredibly vulnerable to long-term health problems and causing you to underperform in aspects of your life.

This is no way to be living. We need to treat mental health just as seriously as we would any illness and need to do something now before it gets worse. But what can we do?

What is Anxiety?

Anxiety is a normal feeling, but it is considered a disorder or problem once the symptoms interfere with an individual's ability to function normally.

Without feelings of anxiety, it's likely that our ancestors would not have survived very long or that the human race would have been so successful. For our ancestors, anxiety at the sight of a prowling lion sent adrenaline through their systems, which prompted the "fight or flight" response and helped them to live another day.

Today, anxiety remains a common emotion, but the focus is often shifted to more abstract and usually more trivial issues than prowling predators. Bill payments, worries over jobs, loss, or divorce all stimulate feelings of uncertainty and anxiety. Even relatively mundane things such as going out, being late, and tests can cause anxiety to flare up. The emotion becomes a disorder when we fail to control our worries and concerns; some people are able to do this more effectively than others. For those with normal anxiety responses, the emotion is quickly dispelled, but for those with an anxiety disorder, this is much harder, and the condition can affect every aspect of their daily lives – in some cases to a crippling extent.

Anxiety is often looked at as the enemy in our culture. The goal is to get rid of it, usually with medication. Anxiety is very bad for your health in so many different ways. It is vital that you take control of your life and conquer the anxiety you might have.

A person experiencing anxiety can certainly manage to cope enough to get through their day, but that anxiety is taking a toll on their life. It's building stress around them, and it can increase the risk of some serious health conditions, including heart attacks, strokes, panic attacks, and much more.

What is PTSD or Post-Traumatic Stress Disorder

Life is unpredictable, and there are chances you

have had some horrible physical or emotional traumas that have left a distressing mark on you. A loved one's death or a horrifying accident is an example. It is possible that just being witness to a situation can cause PTSD. Some of the symptoms include reliving the trauma, responding to a similar situation frantically, or always being apprehensive that it can occur again. You might feel detached or disinterested; far worse, you might become emotionally numb if not attended to.

This can develop once someone has experienced or witnessed something very difficult, violent, or traumatic. They often relive something painful repeatedly, and might be withdrawn emotionally, get angry fast, or have outbursts. The symptoms of PTSD might start right away or could come on years after the incident or incidents. Physical attack, natural disasters, and war are all common triggers of PTSD, and anxious episodes can come on with no signs or warnings.

This condition is usually triggered by real events in life; these are usually serious and very frightening. They include involvement in road accidents, violent assault (including sexual assault), witnessing violent events, military combat, witnessing or being involved in terrorist attacks or severe natural disasters. Not everyone involved in traumatic events develops the condition, but estimates suggest that up to 30 % of those involved in traumatic situations will develop PTSD.

What is Depression

Depression is caused by changes in life circumstances, grief, stress, alterations in hormone levels, medical conditions, and several other traumatic and overwhelming demands of life. These factors alter the brain chemistry. The onset of depression and its expression differs among people. How people deal with grief is, in part, influenced by their genetic patterns.

Depression is linked to the state of our heart, our heart is linked to our emotions or feelings, and our emotions or feelings are linked to our thoughts. If you feel overwhelmed or anxious about a situation or unforeseen circumstances have made a significant impact in your life, and you don't get the right psychological support or tools to help you, this can have a long-term effect on the state of your heart and mental health. Deferred hope and storing anxiety in our hearts can weigh us down, causing us to experience depression. This is why the mental illness approach to depression can keep us stuck in a cycle of depression because it doesn't give us hope that we will ever be able to move forward and live a life free from depression. We need to take a new approach when providing therapy to people who suffer from depression, and that approach is giving them the strategies to improve their mental health, which provides them with hope instead of teaching people they will always have a mental illness.

Often we focus solely on our minds when it comes to depression. Yes, our minds are essential, but our hearts, emotions, and thoughts are all interrelated, and we must pay attention to all of these precious parts of our inner self and physical body. I completely respect the medical field and all the fantastic people who work in that industry. However, the medical field often treats our physical symptoms and diagnoses our situations based on what our physical body is telling us, but how did we get to that state in the first place? When we seek help from a medical doctor, they are not extensively trained in the field of psychological development, and they don't have the time to listen to our most profound thoughts that lead to our emotional issues or the state of our heart. Expecting them to be able to fix depression when the cause isn't a physical issue, will continue to lead us down a road of defeat when it comes to depression.

The physical symptoms of depression are often said to be caused by a chemical imbalance in the brain and are treated with a drug based on this symptom. We can't merely take medication and expect our depression to be healed. The cause must be dealt with if we want our mental health to improve or change permanently. Medication might help to relieve some of the symptoms we are experiencing, but we need to realize medication alone is not going to cure our depression. As a society, we have become lazy and accustomed to fast food convenience expecting all of our answers to be given to us in a prescription. Life can be hard, and sometimes we have to make changes that we might not necessarily want to make. However, if we are going to improve our mental health and live a life free of depression, we need to take action to make choices that are healthy for us as individuals.

If your job, living situation, environment, or relationships are causing you to experience toxic emotions continually, you may have to decide to change the way you are reacting to those circumstances or leave that situation altogether. Our mental health is just as important as our physical health, and we need to be wise in determining what we allow to affect our emotions. If we take this approach to our mental health on a daily basis, this will protect us from experiencing long-term mental health issues.

When we begin to understand ourselves, we will naturally be drawn to the people who are like us, and we can learn to grow into the person we were created to be. We will begin to love ourselves, even when the people around us are not showing love towards us.

If you're unhappy, maybe you don't know who you are, and you are trying to fit into an environment that doesn't understand you? When we try to put a puzzle together, and we put a piece in the wrong place, it doesn't fit, right? We need the right parts in the right areas for the puzzle to be completed.

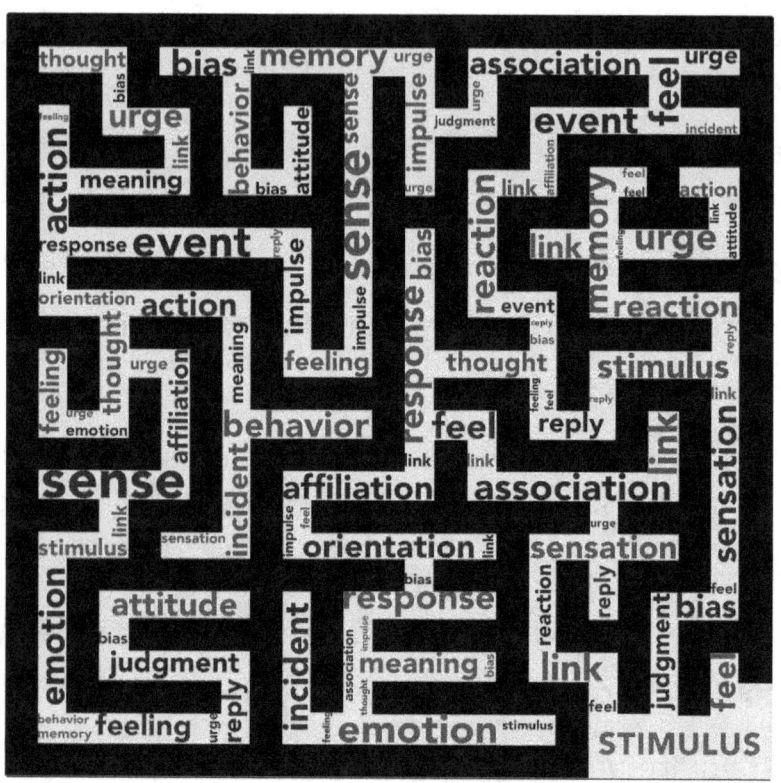

CHAPTER 10
CAUSES OF ANXIETY, DEPRESSION, AND INFLAMMATION

Relationship between inflammation, depression, and anxiety

There is developing proof that inflammation can intensify or even offer ascent to burdensome side effects. The inflammatory response is a key part of our insusceptible framework. At the point when our bodies are attacked by microscopic organisms, infections, poisons, or parasites, the insusceptible framework initiates cells, proteins, and tissues, including the cerebrum, to assault these intruders. The principal technique is to stamp the harmed body parts so that we can give more consideration to them. Nearby inflammation makes the harmed parts red, swollen, and hot. At the point when the damage isn't confined, at that point, the framework ends up aggravated. These ace inflammatory variables offer ascent to "affliction practices." These incorporate physical, psychological, and social changes. Normally, they wiped out individual encounters languor, weakness, slow response time, psychological impedances, and loss of craving. This star grouping of changes that happen when we are wiped out is versatile. It constrains us to get more rest to mend and stay disconnected so as not to spread diseases.

Be that as it may, a drawn-out inflammatory response can unleash ruin in our bodies and can put us in danger of depression and different sicknesses. There is a lot of proof cementing the connection between inflammation and depression. For instance, markers of inflammation are raised in individuals who experience the ill effects of depression contrasted with non-discouraged ones. Additionally, markers of inflammation can anticipate the seriousness of burdensome manifestations. An investigation that analyzed twins who offer 100 percent of similar qualities found that the twin who had a higher CRP fixation (a proportion of inflammation) was bound to create depression five years after the fact.

Specialists saw that their malignancy and Hepatitis C patients treated with IFN-alpha therapy (increments inflammatory response) likewise experienced depression. This treatment expanded the arrival of genius inflammatory cytokines, which offered ascend to lost hunger, rest aggravation, anhedonia (loss of joy), subjective impedance, and self-destructive ideation. The pervasiveness of depression in these patients was high. These outcomes add assurance to the inflammation story of depression.

Ensuing cautious investigations demonstrated that the expansion in the commonness of depression in patients treated with IFN-alpha was not just in light of the fact that they were wiped out. Utilizing a basic technique for infusing sound subjects with invulnerable framework intruders, specialists discovered higher paces of burdensome side effects during the ones which were presented contrasted with the fake treatment gathering. The subjects who were initiated to have an inflammatory response whined of indications, for example, negative state of mind, anhedonia, rest unsettling influences, social withdrawal, and intellectual weaknesses.

The connection between inflammation and depression is much increasingly strong for patients who don't react to flow antidepressants. Studies have demonstrated that treatment-safe patients will, in general, have raised inflammatory components circling at gauge than the responsive ones. This is clinically significant; a clinician can use a measure like CRP levels, which are a piece of a routine physical, to foresee the restorative response to antidepressants. In one examination, they found that expanded degrees of an inflammation particle preceding treatment anticipated poor response to antidepressants.

There are ecological components that reason inflammation and, in this way, lift hazard for depression: stress, low financial status, or agitated youth. Additionally, a raised inflammatory response prompts expanded affectability to stretch. The impact has been accounted for in numerous investigations in mice. For instance, mice that have gone under ceaseless flighty pressure have more elevated levels of inflammation markers. Strikingly, there are singular contrasts that make a few mice progressively impervious to push, in this way, starting a quieter safe response.

Depression is a heterogeneous disorder. Every patient's battle is extraordinary given their youth, hereditary qualities, and the affectability of their resistant framework, other existing real diseases, and their low status in the public eye. Being on the disadvantageous finish of these measurements bothers our safe framework and causes incessant inflammation. The cerebrum is extremely responsive to these flowing inflammatory markers and starts "infection conduct." When the inflammation is drawn out by stressors or different vulnerabilities, the affliction conduct moves toward becoming a depression.

Reasons for anxiety

Anxiety might be brought about by a state of mind, a physical condition, the effects of medications, or a blend of these. The specialist's underlying assignment is to check whether your anxiety is a manifestation of another ailment.

Current research on Anxiety Disorder

Much research is being done into what causes anxiety disorders. Specialists trust it includes a mix of components, including qualities, diet, and stress.

Investigations of twins recommend that hereditary qualities may assume a job. For instance, an investigation announced in PLoS ONE Trusted Source recommends the RBFOX1 quality might be engaged with the improvement of anxiety-related conditions, for example, summed up anxiety disorder. The creators accept that both hereditary and nongenetic variables have an influence.

Certain pieces of the cerebrum, for example, the amygdala and hippocampus, are additionally being considered. Your amygdala is a little structure somewhere inside your cerebrum that procedures risk. It cautions the remainder of your mind when there are indications of risk. It can trigger a dread and anxiety response. It appears to have an influence on anxiety disorders that include dread of explicit things, for example, felines, honey bees, or suffocating.

Your hippocampus may likewise influence your danger of building up an anxiety disorder. It's a locale of your cerebrum that is associated with putting away recollections of undermining occasions. It seems, by all accounts, to be littler in individuals who've encountered kid misuse or served in battle.

What causes anxiety disorders?

Anxiety is a psychological wellness condition that can cause sentiments of stress, dread, or pressure.

For certain individuals, anxiety can likewise cause fits of anxiety and extraordinary physical side effects, similar to chest torment.

The definite reasons for anxiety disorders are obscure. As indicated by the National Institute of Mental Health, specialists accept that a mix of hereditary and ecological variables may assume a job. Cerebrum science is likewise being concentrated as a conceivable reason. The zones of your mind that control your dread response might be included.

Anxiety disorders frequently happen close by other psychological wellness conditions, for example, substance misuse and depression. Numerous individuals attempt to facilitate the side effects of anxiety by utilizing liquor or different medications. The help these substances give is brief. Liquor, nicotine, caffeine, and different medications can exacerbate an anxiety disorder.

Anxiety disorders are unimaginably normal. They influence an expected 40 million individuals in the United States, as indicated by the Anxiety and Depression Association of America.

What causes anxiety and anxiety disorders can be muddled. Almost certainly, a blend of components, including hereditary qualities and ecological reasons, assume a job. In any case, plainly a few occasions, feelings, or encounters may make side effects of anxiety start or may aggravate them. These components are called triggers.

Anxiety triggers can be distinctive for every individual, except numerous triggers, are normal among individuals with these conditions. A great many people discover they have numerous triggers. Be that as it may, for certain individuals, anxiety assaults can be activated for reasons unknown by any stretch of the imagination.

Therefore, it's imperative to find any anxiety triggers that you may have. Distinguishing your triggers is a significant advance in overseeing them. Continue perusing to find out about these anxiety triggers and what you can do to deal with your anxiety.

What are the anxiety triggers

Health Issues

A wellbeing analysis that is annoying or troublesome, for example, malignancy or a constant sickness, may trigger anxiety or exacerbate it. This kind of trigger is ground-breaking on account of the prompt and individual sentiments it produces.

You can help lessen anxiety brought about by medical problems by being proactive and drawn in with your primary care physician. Conversing with a specialist may likewise be valuable, as they can enable you to figure out how to deal with your feelings around your analysis.

Medications

Certain remedy and over-the-counter (OTC) medications may trigger indications of anxiety. That is on the grounds that dynamic fixings in these medications may make you feel uneasy or unwell. Those emotions can set off a progression of occasions in your brain and body that may prompt extra side effects of anxiety.

Prescriptions that may trigger anxiety include:

- Birth control pills
- Cough and blockage medications
- Weight misfortune medications

Converse with your PCP about how these medications make you feel and search for an elective that doesn't trigger your anxiety or decline your side effects.

Caffeine

Numerous individuals depend on their morning cup of joe to wake up; however, it may really trigger or exacerbate anxiety. As per one investigation in 2010Trusted Source, individuals with frenzy disorder and social anxiety disorder are particularly touchy to the anxiety-inciting effects of caffeine.

Work to curtail your caffeine admission by substituting noncaffeinated alternatives at whatever point conceivable.

Skipping Suppers

When you don't eat, your glucose may drop. That can prompt anxious hands and a thundering stomach. It can likewise trigger anxiety.

Eating adjusted suppers is significant for some reasons. It furnishes you with vitality and significant supplements. In the event that you can't set aside a few minutes for three suppers per day, solid tidbits are an extraordinary method to anticipate low glucose, sentiments of nervousness or fomentation, and anxiety. Keep in mind, and nourishment can influence your disposition.

Negative Reasoning

Your mind controls quite a bit of your body, and that is positively valid with anxiety. When you're vexed or baffled, the words you state to yourself can trigger more prominent sentiments of anxiety.

On the off chance that you will, in general, utilize a lot of negative words when considering yourself, figuring out how to refocus your language and sentiments when you start down this way is useful. Working with an advisor can be fantastically useful with this procedure.

Budgetary Concerns

Stresses over setting aside cash or having an obligation can trigger anxiety. Sudden bills or cash fears are triggers, as well.

Figuring out how to deal with these sorts of triggers may need looking for expert support, for example, from a monetary guide. Feeling you have a buddy and a guide in the process may facilitate your worry.

Gatherings or Get-Togethers

In the event that a room brimming with outsiders doesn't seem like fun, you're not the only one. Occasions that expect you to make casual chitchat or associate with individuals you don't know can trigger sentiments of anxiety, which might be analyzed as a social anxiety disorder.

To help facilitate your stresses or unease, you can continually bring along a friend when conceivable. But at the same time, it's critical to work with an expert to discover methods for dealing with stress that make these occasions increasingly sensible in the long haul.

Struggle

Relationship issues, contentions, differences — these contentions would all be able to trigger or compound anxiety. On the off chance that contention especially triggers you, you may need to learn compromise systems. Additionally, converse with an advisor or another emotional well-being master to figure out how to deal with the sentiments these contentions cause.

Stress

Day by day stressors like congested driving conditions or missing your train can cause anybody anxiety. Yet, long haul or constant pressure can prompt long haul anxiety and compounding manifestations, just as other medical issues.

Stress can likewise prompt practices like skipping dinners, drinking liquor, or not getting enough rest. These elements can trigger or intensify anxiety, as well.

Treating and avoiding pressure regularly requires getting the hang of methods for dealing with stress. A specialist or advocate can enable you to figure out how to perceive your wellsprings of stress and handle them when they become overpowering or hazardous.

Open Occasions or Exhibitions

Open talking, talking before your chief, performing in a challenge, or even simply perusing so anyone might hear is a typical trigger of anxiety. In the event that your activity or diversions require this, your primary care physician or advisor can work with you to learn approaches to be increasingly agreeable in these settings.

Additionally, uplifting comments from companions and associates can enable you to feel increasingly good and sure.

Individual Triggers

These triggers might be hard to distinguish, yet a psychological well-being authority is prepared to enable you to recognize them. These may start with a smell, a spot, or even a tune. Individual triggers remind you, either intentionally or unknowingly, of an awful memory or awful accident in your life. People with post-awful pressure disorder (PTSD) as often as possible experience anxiety triggers from ecological triggers.

Distinguishing individual triggers may require some serious energy, yet it's significant so you can figure out how to conquer them.

CHAPTER 11
POWER OF YOUR BODY WITH SELF-HELP EXERCISES AND TECHNIQUES

Exercise

Exercise is a necessary part of healing from chronic pain. You don't have to become an active bodybuilder or an athlete, but some degree of body movement is highly desirable to prevent chronic pain. Body movements release the "stuck" energy in our body and ensure a smooth flow of energy to prevent any pain.

Exercising is a great way to reduce your anxiety whether you wake up earlier in the morning before you have to go to work and go for a run or if you can when you get home from work to go out and jog around the block.

Also, if you do exercise more, this will help with your self-esteem. Exercising will make you healthier, and you will feel better about yourself. If you are worried about your health and it is making your anxiety worse, get out there and do some exercises.

You don't even have to leave your house, and you could just find an exercise DVD and start doing some exercise from your own living room. To really help lower anxiety, it is a good idea for each time you exercise to be sure it is for 30 minutes or more. Studies have shown that it takes about thirty minutes for your anxiety to lower when exercising.

If you don't want to exercise alone, grab a friend to do this activity with you. This will make you happy, and you can have someone to talk to about the things you are anxious about. It's great to have someone to let all of your feelings out to who can help you. Healthy exercise has some surprising implications for those with anxiety disorders and other psychological conditions, including depression. The mechanisms by which exercise and mental health are related are not fully understood, but many medical experts around the world now acknowledge that exercise has a major impact on a wide range of psychological conditions. It is even now believed that exercise can be as effective at combating depression as many commonly prescribed drugs.

Short bursts of activity a few times a day are the type of exercise that experts recommend. A brisk walk lasting only ten minutes is believed to be enough to raise your emotional state for a couple of hours. For those with anxiety disorders, it can be hard to get out and about on occasion. For some, with severe conditions, it can seem impossible. Exercise, however, will really help to improve your emotional state and take your mind off the anxiety. Use the following tips to increase your chances of successfully incorporating exercise into your life.

Moderate level intensity exercise is recommended as perfect for improving your physical health and also your mental health. This includes; walking briskly, cycling, jogging, or swimming. Walking and jogging should not need any investment, and if you're uncomfortable alone, partner up with a friend or relative. Ideally, buddy up with someone who is addressing the same issues or has a good understanding of them, for extra support.

When we exercise, the brain releases endorphins or "feel-good" chemicals that are responsible for the "high" that many people feel during and after exercise. Another benefit of exercise for those with depression is that it lends purpose and structure to each day. Outdoor exercise has been shown to be especially effective for lifting mood.

Regular exercise can help maintain a healthy weight, which can be a problem in depressed people. Exercise promotes overall wellbeing, including heart health and a toned, more muscular body. The weight-bearing aspects of exercise prevent the body from losing bone mass and decrease the risk of osteoporosis, a particular benefit for women.

People who suffer from anxiety may not be interested in exercise. When someone is overwhelmed by the stress of everyday life, working out seems less than appealing. However, research shows that exercise plays an important role in reducing anxiety symptoms.

While exercise has been clinically proven to reduce anxiety and improve mood, it can also treat a number of other health problems. Health issues can be a major anxiety trigger, and easing the symptoms of those ailments can reduce anxiety symptoms further.

In addition, exercising can help people relax. When a person exercises, their body releases hormones that produce a calming effect. Exercise also increases body temperature, which can be very relaxing. Working up a sweat is tiring, but it's a great way to calm down.

Speed Walking

Speed walking, more often referred to as power walking or race walking, is a technique of walking at a rapid pace. Walking is a great alternative to running and is oftentimes much easier and more accessible to a greater variety of people. Walking provides all of the aerobic benefits of running while steering clear of many of the injuries associated with high-impact techniques of running. The activity of walking at an increased rate, then walking "normally" can help participants lose weight, tone their muscles, and also increase their mood.

Not only is speed walking valuable for the muscles and joints, but it also reinforces overall health.

Stretching

Stretching is something everyone should do on a regular basis, and those with chronic back pain will benefit most from stretching the soft the muscles, ligaments, and tendons in and around the spine.

It is a fact that when motion is limited, the back becomes stiff, which can result in more pain. Those who suffer from chronic back pain need to stretch regularly and perform appropriate stretching movements to benefit from sustained and long-term relief from the increased motion.

One top recommendation for dealing with chronic pain is by getting regular exercise. Exercise will help with different types of pain, from helping with arthritis by getting your body moving to boost your mood when you have pain from Crohn's or fibromyalgia.

Yoga for Chronic Pain

Yoga can also be defined as an art based on the harmonizing system of developing the mind, body, and soul. By practicing Yoga every day, you will not only explore your true self or your inner self but also develop the feeling that you are one with nature and environment. Yoga caters to the overall well-being of the body and focuses mainly on developing a relationship with the natural world around us.

Pain is not just influenced by physical injury or illness. It is also greatly affected by our thoughts, anxiety, trauma, stress, and emotions. Stress and pain are closely interrelated - you may experience pain when stressed, and stress can also increase the intensity of the pain. When there is increased stress, the breathing becomes heavier, erratic, and ragged.

The mood is also altered, along with some tension and tightening of the muscles. These symptoms of chronic pain can even increase the toxins in the body and decrease oxygen levels.

Yoga addresses these problems effectively as it involves the techniques of deep breathing and meditation, which helps in the absorption of much-needed oxygen and also in the relaxation of mind and body. These breathing techniques ensure that the muscles of the lungs, diaphragm, back, and abdomen are worked out. When the muscles are loose and relaxed, they can help in releasing the built-up tension in the body and facilitate the proper flow of energy throughout. Stress and anxiety levels will also reduce gradually.

Yoga or simple stretching are simple practices that should be applied to everyday life to reduce the tension of stress and keep the muscles in proper working order. There are specific stretches that can focus on problem areas such as the neck or lower back. These stretches can be assigned from a personal trainer, massage therapist, or physiotherapist. Yoga can be enjoyed at home or in a studio with several other participants. There are many forms of yoga ranging from hatha yoga to hot yoga. The focus in yoga is on breath control, meditation, stretching, and balance. Not all forms of yoga are spiritual with chants and mantras if you don't feel comfortable with that form of practice.

Exercise, in general, is good for chronic pain, but specific exercises, especially certain yoga positions, helps to decrease some types of pain, like shoulder or neck pain.

And the relaxation techniques you will learn can teach you how to manage the different types of chronic pain more effectively.

If you are considering trying yoga techniques for your chronic pain, you need to consider the style of yoga you will do.

While all forms of **yoga** can be beneficial for your body, mind, and spirit, certain exercises are actually directed towards people who are struggling with chronic pain.

There are multiple yoga poses or asanas, and a different stance can be used. Individuals with chronic pain should begin with a slow-paced, gentle yoga pose. Benefits of yoga include improved ability to handle stress, feeling more relaxed throughout the day, and improvements in sleep quality. Studies have proven that yoga is helpful to prevent fibromyalgia, among other chronic pain conditions.

Massage Therapy

Massage therapy has become overwhelmingly popular, and rightfully so, in addition to feeling good, it has a number of health benefits. Massage therapy is wonderful for any type of pain, be it chronic, acute, or simply from fatigue, work, and tension. There are various massage therapies available to meet all types of needs, including Shiatsu, Swedish, hot oil, and deep tissue.

Massage has also been used as a natural anxiety remedy for ages; it may be as simple as rubbing your neck gently, but whichever the case, you are massaging your way to calm nerves. The benefits of any massage therapy are many amongst them, stress relief, relaxation, lowers blood pressure, lowers tension build in the muscles, and it also improves deeper breathing. As the book unfolds, I will discuss therapeutic massage as a natural remedy for anxiety disorders; in this case, it will be much deeper and more precise.

A skilled and trained massage therapist will know exactly what to do once the pain problem is explained. Massage also does wonders for fatigue and stress, both of which are known exasperate pain and both of which go hand in hand with arthritis and other chronic pain conditions. It can also help to calm anxiety, which often afflicts those who suffer from chronic pain.

If you can afford it, get a massage regularly, weekly, or even twice per week. Physical therapists and chiropractors also offer therapeutic massage so that it may be covered under medical insurance.

There are also some great electronic massagers on the market that are great options. These include mobile units, spot massage products that target the neck or specific areas. There are also strap onto chair units that offer shiatsu for the entire back, and many come with a heat option.

The most significant health benefit of massage is that it provides the sensation of touch, which is critical in both early childhood development and overall adult health. Levels of somatotropin, or human growth hormone, correlate directly with the amount of physical contact you receive.

Massage also cues relaxation in your nervous system. One of the biggest benefits of massage is that it feels great, especially if you're in pain. Nerves that carry information about the sensation of touch to the brain are more heavily myelinated than the nerves that carry information about pain, so touch information travels faster than pain information. This is why you instinctively rub the skin around a painful area; the touch sensation temporarily drowns out the pain sensation, and you're given a brief moment of relief.

Massage also feels good because it temporarily reduces muscle tension. Pressing on tight muscles lengthens them in the same way that gentle prolonged static stretching does, and after an hour or so of this manual lengthening, you may stand up feeling like your muscles are made of jelly. If your massage therapist applies a great deal of pressure, your stretch reflex may be activated immediately, making you feel tight and sore soon after a massage. A good rule of thumb is that if you feel pain during a massage, you're probably going to feel some soreness afterward as well. While it can be difficult or awkward at the moment, it's better to ask your massage therapist to press more gently than to suffer the consequences. It is absolutely not necessary to apply a painful amount of pressure to reap the benefits of a massage. Moreover, if you're in pain, a deep massage can increase and prolong your pain by making your muscles tighter.

Lastly, massage temporarily softens connective tissues, which increases flexibility and range of motion. Tendons, ligaments, fascia (which surrounds, supports, and separates structures of the body), and scar tissue (which forms to heal an injury) are all made of collagen fibers arranged in varying patterns and densities. As muscles become habitually tighter and movement decreases, connective tissues also respond by tightening. Movement and heat can make these collagen structures more flexible and fluid.

For people with chronic pain, the most beneficial aspect of massage maybe that it lowers stress, thereby reducing the sensation of pain and reactivity of the nervous system. A massage by itself is not enough to change deeply learned habitual movements or your resting level of muscle tension. The sensory awareness that can be gained through massage is valuable, but if it isn't followed by actual motor education in the form of voluntary movement, little lasting progress will be made. You must actively retrain your nervous system, and you can't do that with massage alone.

Brain Balance

First, you have to make sure your brain is balanced. Without a balanced nervous system, your efforts to eliminate chronic pain will be wasted. Causes of Brain Imbalance Many things can cause brain imbalances. Most common are head injury and exposure to electromagnetic radiation from personal wireless devices.

Things that increase brain imbalance risk factors include:

- Using Bluetooth devices and cell phones, walkie talkie, using desktop and laptop computers, and iPad.
- Eating processed foods that might have MSG
- Consuming drinks containing artificial sweeteners, drinking fluoridated water.

- Leading a stressful life
- Not getting enough quality sleep
- Brain balancing using affirmations

Studies show that when the thymus gland is balanced, both hemispheres of the brain also remain balanced and lower chronic pain. The nice thing about the affirmations is that they don't cost you anything; you just have to repeat the affirmations regularly throughout the day to keep your brain balance. You need to "feel" the words to get full benefits.

Following is a list of daily affirmations:

- I have faith, gratitude, trust, love, and courage.
- I'm modest, and I'm humble and tolerant.
- I'm clean and good, and I deserved to be loved
- I'm content and tranquil
- I have forgiveness in my heart
- My life energy is high, and life is full of love

Brain Balancing Music

Brain balancing music encourages a balanced nervous system and balances both hemispheres of the brain. Brain balancing music uses three coordinated methods: "Primordial Sounds," "Brainwave Entrainment," and "multi-layered music" to bring the mind-body into a deeply relaxed and balanced state. You have to listen to music on a daily basis to maintain your brain balanced. Brain balance is crucial for the health and healing of chronic pain.

Avoid GMO foods

GMO or genetically modified organisms are introduced to our diets over the past decade. As of this writing, the GMO foods are not labeled in the U. S. So, the average American's unconsciously consuming GMO rich canola, sugar beets, corn, soy, and cottonseed oil. GMO foods can cause all sorts of gastrointestinal symptoms, allergies, weight gain, and immune problems. Avoiding GMO foods can reduce or even eliminate many health problems, including chronic pain.

Emotional Freedom Techniques

This amazing technique deals swiftly with all sorts

of emotional pain and has an infinite number of applications. EFT has been around for quite a while and is now used in many hospitals and psych units throughout the world by professional psychologists and psychiatrists who are continuing to get very positive results with severe emotional pain and trauma.

There is no doubt strong emotions can be very painful things, and it is now recognized that emotion follows thought. This is why psychiatrists spend years talking about trauma, trying to uncover triggers and thoughts that cause bad feelings, depression, phobias, and the like.

What you do is tap lightly on each of them. You get used to doing this very quickly, and when you have been using EFT for a while, you can just do a few taps here and there, maybe on your collarbone or under your eye, for rapid relief.

EFT is a great way to deal with all fear though you will have to be thorough. Really take a look at all the different aspects of that fear and treat each one with a very specific opening statement.

Emotional Freedom Technique (EFT) or tapping requires that you tap specific acupressure points on the torso, hands, and on the head in order to clear energy blocks caused by negative emotions and feelings. Generally, tapping involves two stages. In the first stage, you are tapping to express negative emotions. This stage of tapping will last as long as you have an emotional charge, continual tapping will bring that charge down to a minimal level.

The second stage includes reframing the condition positively where you choose a positive emotion or thought to replace the negative ones. The cool thing is you can't tap incorrectly; your intention is enough to make it work correctly. Even without tapping the right acupressure points, you will still release the negative energy from your body. Basic EFT instructions:

Choose a negative emotion or feeling you wish to clear based on a situation that is troubling you. For example, you might be angry at your neighbor Tom for letting his dog poop in your backyard.

When you feel your emotional charge has dropped significantly and want to move on to the positive rounds, then tap all the acupressure points again and review your state of feelings. For example, as you tap, you might say, "I choose to be open," "I choose forgiveness," "I choose to let go and move on," *etc.*

Cultivating a Positive Attitude

The easiest way I know to create a positive attitude is to count your blessings. I know, I know, that may sound like old hat, you've tried that a hundred times, you think there's nothing to be thankful for, but look closely, chunk down and start really small.

Now do that three times a day. It only takes moments. You can write them down if you wish. First thing in the morning, lunchtime and before bed. Make it a rule and do it for at least a week.

First of all, concentrate on small things, then you will find them extending out, past the current moment. Remember, start small, if you have beautiful, strong nails, list those, if you like the way your old slippers keep your feet snuggly warm, list those. Become aware of the tiniest pleasures throughout the day and mentally add them to your list.

So, the goal is to create an attitude of gratefulness for what you DO have, and in this way, you open the floodgates for a whole lot more of the same. Whatever your beliefs on the subject, it is an inescapable fact that like attracts like, whether that is misery or joy, so you may as well choose joy!

Visualization and Setting Goals

Visualization and setting goals are important. You should have one big goal – to fully heal and return to normal, or an even better life – and some small milestones you will set for yourself. Visualizing a life where you are pain-less and is free to do whatever you want can help in cementing your determination to heal. This will also keep you up when the emotionally-taxing treatment brings you a bit down. By setting a final goal at the end of smaller goals, the big one feels easier. This is achieved by slowly traversing through the smaller goals one by one. Set a daily or weekly goal and visualize what you will be able to think and do by the end of that time period. Always give yourself some time to feel the celebration of your accomplishment for every milestone. Not only will it give you a needed break in your climb towards betterment, but you will also feel more encouraged to go on and reach the final goal.

Guided imagery or creative visualization, as it is commonly called, is another alternative therapy that can be used in pain management. This method involves focusing the imagination on certain positive events or behaviors that you would like to occur in the future. The principle behind this practice is that the mind and the body are connected, and they influence each other. The emotional trauma associated with some physical injuries and events can be replaced by these self suggestions, positive images, and imaginary creative techniques.

Many researchers have stated that visualization is one of the most effective and powerful tools of change. It can have a great positive impact on the patient if guided correctly. Visualization can be done independently or under another's guidance. But most researchers opine that it is more effective when somebody else guides you through the process as you respond more quickly to the guidance of an external voice.

There are numerous ways to start the process of visualization. If you are practicing it independently, there are many CD's available online and in retail outlets that can guide you through the process.

By doing this, the brain starts to respond to the inputs given in the form of two-dimensional images.

Then the brain sends out the signal for the body to relax. Therefore, by imagining the situation where you don't feel any pain, the body relaxes as the brain starts responding to those stimuli. This technique is very effective in treating different types of health issues, both physical and emotional.

Visualization should ideally be performed in a quiet area where you will not be disturbed or distracted. It is best to keep the lighting dim or even maintain total darkness - that generally works best for visualization. Each of the sessions may last from 20 minutes to an hour, and you may start feeling slightly positive changes from the very first session.

Music Therapy

It should create a gentle and relaxing response in the person listening to the music, which, if done right, can help them reduce their pain or at least help them handle it better.

With just a little research, you can experiment with music therapy on your own, or seek out a licensed musical therapist who has gone through a training program.

Music therapy offers numerous health benefits, but

it is frequently used for physical and mental pain management.

It helps to relieve stress and anxiety, which is often exasperated by pain, as well as giving you a mood boost when you are experiencing chronic pain.

Your music therapy program might include listening to music or getting you involved in making music, writing songs, or just singing along to songs.

There are several reasons to give it a try.

- You may not need to use as much pain medication, which can cause other body issues, can become addictive, and eventually stop working.

- If you find it is helping, add it to your anti-pain arsenal, as it is a good, ongoing therapy that can help with long-term pain management.

- The fact that it can reduce stress and help your body relax is often why it often works for chronic pain management.

- This will help improve your overall quality of life - naturally.

- Find a professional to learn more about music therapy if you would like to explore this natural method for helping with your chronic pain.

Comfort yourself

Comfort and give advice to yourself as if you're helping your best friend or a close family. You are your greatest friend and your closest family, after all, just as you are your worst enemy. It works both ways, you know. Of course, such an activity that requires clarity of thought and focus of your mind requires that you, yourself have identified what exactly is wrong. So dig in and help that pain-filled, trembling you inside that darkened interior of your heart.

Letting Go

It is very painful to blame yourself for something that you have no control over. It has been one of the leading causes of chronic pain symptoms and are usually either self-imposed or are drilled into them all throughout a significant period of time. It could also be an experience long gone in the past that no one can do anything about anymore. In such cases, letting go would be the best option. One cannot totally forget memories, especially those that are heavy enough to cause impacts that affect you physically in the present. But they can be accepted, acknowledged, and regarded as valuable stepping stones for the current you to reach where you are now. Don't endanger the future for something that happened in the past. Let them be your inspiration, your motivation to keep moving forward and up, instead of taking them with you like shackles that remind you of the pain. Don't live in the past, gradually move on into the present, and be hopeful for your future.

Biofeedback

Biofeedback is a special technique that helps people to improve their health conditions by training them to control certain involuntary processes of the body. Using the biofeedback mechanism, the individual learns to change his physiological activity in order to improve health conditions and performance levels.

You may think biofeedback is not a self-help technique to eliminate chronic pain, but it is really an effective method. Biofeedback is helpful for everything from gastric distress, high blood pressure, migraine headache, anxiety, sleep disorders, and muscle pains. Biofeedback is generally done under the supervision of a health professional, but with a little training, you can do it yourself. Basically, biofeedback involves listening to a relaxation tape and having a small electrode taped to one of your fingers.

Biofeedback sessions can take 15 to 30 minutes, and during that time, you will be using guided imagery and relaxation breathing. While you are practicing relaxing methods, you can see your heart rate or skin temperature on the monitor.

The therapy involves attaching electrodes to the skin, which displays the results to a connected monitor, and this is the information that is used to help control your involuntary functions. There is no exact evidence on how the biofeedback technique works, but many experiments conducted by researchers have reported that it gives relief from stress and helps the body to relax, which is vital for maintaining good health.

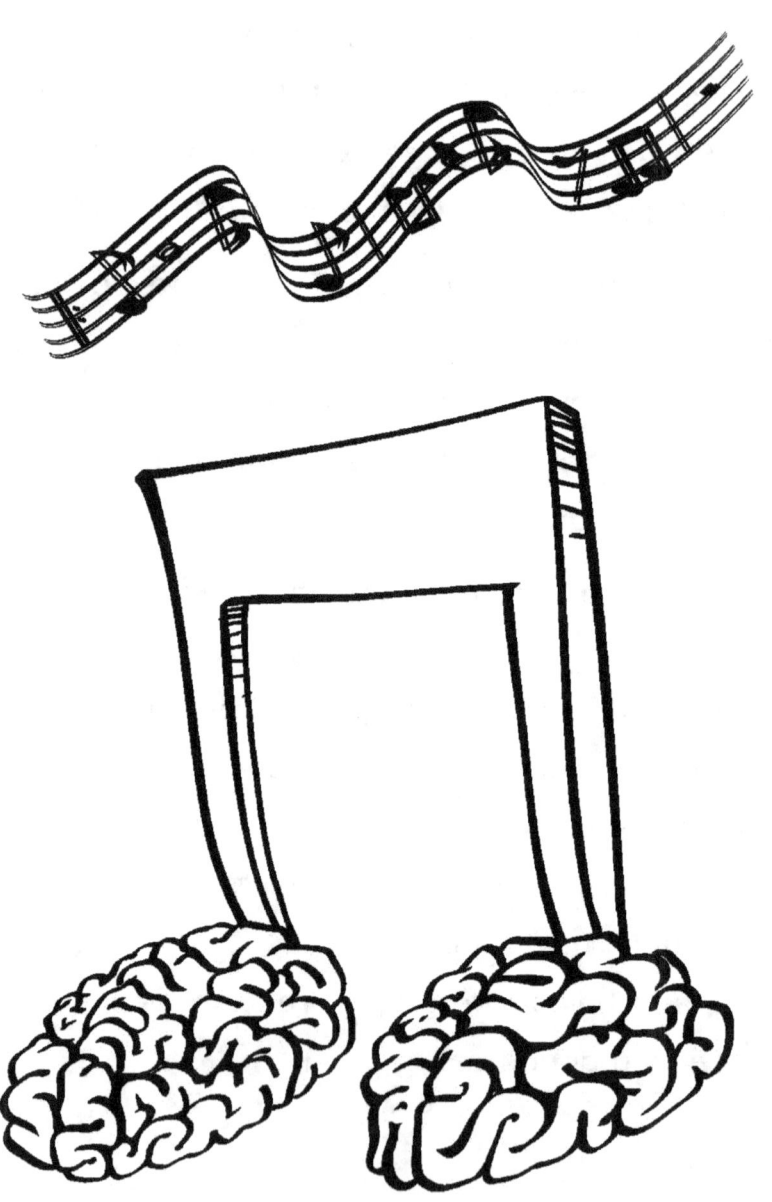

CHAPTER 12
MUSIC

The Role of Music in the Polyvagal Theory

Music paints a picture of the world around us and uploads it directly to our brain. It can take us from scared, frozen in fear, to energized and activated. It can make us sad or happy, raise us to heights of triumph or drag us down to the depths of defeat and sorrow. It makes sense then that music can have a direct impact on our perceived state of being as affected by our vagus nerve.

A musical score with discordant notes in a minor key, an unsteady rhythm, all sends signals of danger to our brain. In the same way, a piece of music that is either very low pitched or, in contrast is very high pitched can send danger signals. Perhaps this is why we use deep-toned sounds for foghorns as warning signals, but we also react to a baby's high-pitched scream as a sign that immediate parental action is required.

Music that runs too fast can make us feel uneasy as if we are in danger of missing important information, but music that runs too slow can give the impression that the message is not coming across quickly enough.

Not much study has been done surrounding music and how it may or may not impact our natural sense of safety, but in August 2015, one article was published that may shed some insight on this process.

The conductors of the experiment wanted to find out what brought on the most sense of safety: silence, sounds of nature, or music. In essence, they wanted to find out if music could trigger a sense of safety.

Their study came away with several conclusions and some surprising findings, one of which being that a cappella music was seen as slightly more dangerous than straight instrumental music. Their guess about this finding was that perhaps it was because voice music carries a bit more variability and unpredictability than the instrumental would have. Perhaps also it could be explained by the notion of human voices raised in unison brings with it a sense of urgency or a call to action, unlike non-voiced instrumental music.

One of the two main focuses of the study was to find out if music holds fewer dangerous signals than nature sounds and silence. The study showed that yes, music was seen as an indicator of safety. This may tell us that music provides an information system that tells the body things about its environment. Simple music without much movement was also seen as more dangerous or stress-inducing than music more complex and faster. Music that was too fast was seen as a stressor or danger signal as well.

It was interesting to note that each person's optimal speed and intensity of the music was different.

Through this, we can see that music could be an important part of overcoming trauma and sustaining a healthy mind and body relationship.

Music has a direct impact on the cranial muscles of the face, meaning the music itself helps to stimulate the vagus nerve and teaches our body how to react to the world around us.

We can also use music to bring us into a healthier state of mind. With today's technology, you can find music to fit every need simply by doing a simple search in your internet browser.

Think of how music can help soothe the mind of an autistic person, offering order and structure, and perhaps a sense of safety in the midst of a world that they see as bombarding them with too much chaotic information at all times.

That same sort of soothing can be for you too.

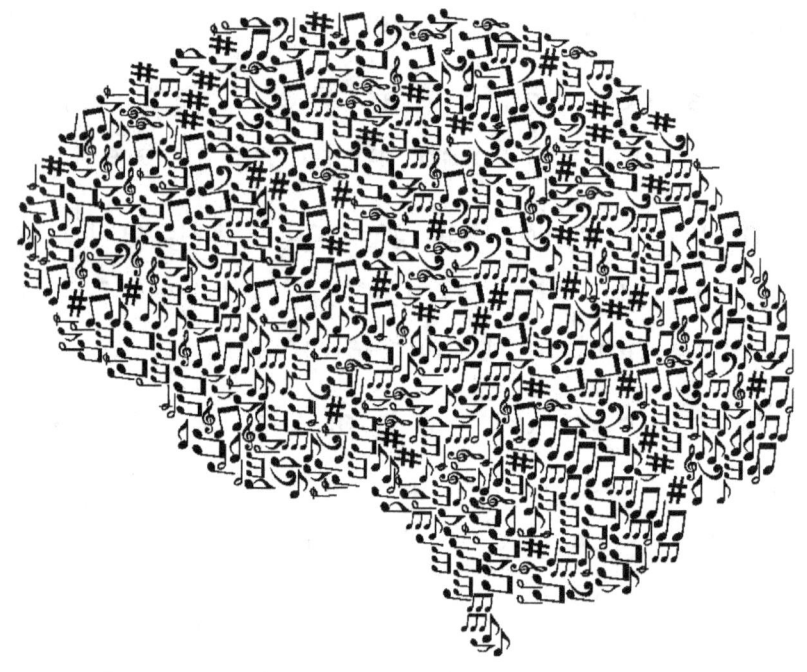

CHAPTER 13
SOCIAL MEDIA

Vagus Nerve and Social Media

Social media is a part of our lives now. There is no going back, and I doubt that we ought even to try. Social media says to our brains that we are being social, but are we? Are we connecting on that neurological level?

Recent studies have found that higher use of social media actually correlates with higher feelings of isolation among teenagers. This tells me that being on social media does not always tell your body that you are in a community of other people, that you are being accepted and welcomed in and responded to.

Sometimes people intentionally inflate their followers or their friends' list on whatever social media platform they prefer. They are trying to create a crowd in the hopes that the more numbers they see, the more they will feel as if they are in a community with other people. Contrary to their intentions, all this does is inflate their isolation. The numbers do not have arms to reach out, and subconsciously we realize this.

Can we have meaningful relationships online? Yes, I believe so. There are anecdotes all around us of people who have deep and satisfying relationships with people they have met online. Those friends are just as many friends as people we know offline. The difference is that in trying to create a crowd, we wind up relying on numbers rather than a real conversation. This is part of the story we tell ourselves again. When a person begins to rely on the numbers, they see revolving around their social media platform, and then the social connection becomes all about a shallow reward-based system. Make a post or share a picture that gets likes, and then interpret that as the reward, creating an entire relationship around the clicking of a button.

As much as it is true online, you can feel terribly alone standing in a crowd of people who are physically present with you. Having a crowd around you means nothing if no one is there with you, being present with you, and joining in with you. Even a stranger who pauses to notice you will be enough to ease some of that loneliness when in a physical crowd.

Just as in your offline life, having a few close friends who really understand you and take time to talk and interact with you on a deeper basis is what will create that feeling of community that you long for. The problem with social media that I see is that it relies so heavily on numbers rather than any meaningful connection.

Secondarily, another problem with social media is that you can put up an image of yourself that is only a partial image, or is airbrushed, sometimes literally. What you put on those social media platforms can be only the best of yourself, only the brightest, only the perfect. And when people respond positively to that, you are unconsciously teaching yourself that people only like the best parts of you. This does not create a trusting relationship, and we instinctively know it. This creates a social connection based on an image, a fake image, and that is a very lonely thing indeed.

You can change this. You can create an online sense of community as well as an offline one. I do believe it is better to have that offline connection, though as well. Don't isolate yourself from those physically with you. We all need that physical interaction, so do not deprive yourself of that. We are finding out that our very neurons cry out for that connection with other people.

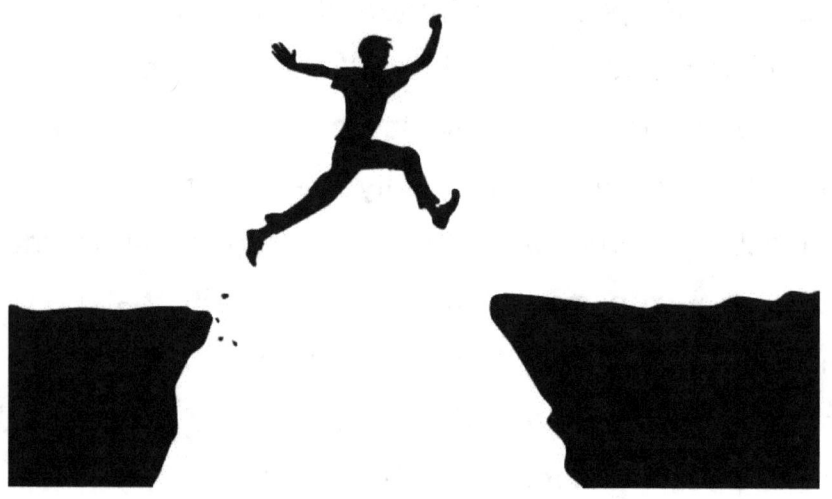

CHAPTER 14
CREATE SAFETY

Safe and Social

After all this, your sense of well-being and safety is up to you. You can choose to reach out to get help from others. You can surround yourself with things that help you stay in that optimal state. You can create the story that you tell yourself.

Creating safety around yourself will bring you back into a more balanced perspective on life, and to a place of more healthful living.

Be creative: write. You do not have to be good at it; you just need to write. Put the feelings down on paper and let them speak for themselves now. Leave those feelings there as you are writing them down. The physical act of writing can have a deep impact on your sense of safety, allowing an outlet for the muscles to release some of that energy.

Find a focus – distract yourself from the anxiety by looking for something specific in your environment. Look for a pebble, a leaf, a flower, find the clouds, or look for something blue. Be creative. Become a hunter of that object or color.

The human voice can sometimes kickstart us into our ventral system. Listen to a podcast or an inspirational message. Listen to the soothing voice of a narrator reading a favorite book or a new book we have never read.

Get grounded: focus on the floor under your feet, the armrests under your arms, the seat under your seat. Feel the breeze on your face; let your body feel cold or hot, feel the hair move on your head. Concentrate on what your eyes see, focus in on what your ears are hearing, identify some smells in your environment.

Remember that the nervous system's automatic responses require movement. The need to move is built into us, and so listen to your body. Accept what your body is telling you. Let your body respond to that need but redirect it to a safe activity.

When we create safety for ourselves, we will be better equipped to create safety for those around us as well.

CHAPTER 15
MEDITATION TO ACTIVATE THE VAGUS NERVE

When we activate the vagus nerve, we are going to be doing a lot of great things for our bodies. We are going to help reduce high blood pressure, sharpen our memory, fight inflammation, sleep better, overcome anxiety as well as depression, reduce our allergies, reduce our stress levels, start sprouting new brain cells, turn off the fight or flight response so that we can relax and so much more.

Because there are so many benefits to activating the vagus nerve, it is important for us to make sure that we are doing it properly. There are many ways for us to activate and stimulate the vagus nerve, and we can incorporate them into our everyday lives.

What is Meditation?

Meditation, like exercising, is a skill. It is something that you will have to learn how to do, and it is something that you will get better at over time.

Meditation is very popular right now because people have started to recognize the benefits. They no longer buy into the stigma that it is new age or strange. There are certain circles that still feel that meditation is something that only hippies or monks do, but the majority of people today can see the benefits. You see, anyone can meditate. You don't have to believe in a certain deity or have specific political beliefs, or even be a monk. It does not matter who you are; if you meditate, you will see the benefits.

While it is a very popular technique to use today, many people really don't know what it is. Some people think of meditation as a deep state of concentration when others think of meditation; they think about a peaceful state of mind. They focus on the idea of slowing the mind down in order to get some relief from the stress that they are facing. This is not really what meditation is. You see, we can never stop our minds from being active. Instead, we need to think of meditation as a state of mind. It is an awareness.

You see, we can all be in this state at any point in our day. We do not have to be sitting in a specific position, thinking a specific thought, or focusing on a specific thing. We can experience meditation while we are working, driving, or sitting outside.

Meditation is not concentrating on a certain idea or object for a specified amount of time. This, instead, is visualization. Meditation is not a loss of control. You are not going to hear voices or sounds that are not there, and you are not going to see things that are not there are losing control of your bodily movements.

Meditation is not an exercise. It does not have anything to do with deep breathing, although the two can be used together, and meditation does not require mental effort. You do not have to sit and focus on meditating. Instead, you can focus on other tasks while meditating at the same time. In fact, as I am writing this book, I am practicing meditation.

Benefits of Meditation

1. Meditation is going to provide you with many benefits, which is why so many people are taking notice of it today. They are finding that it helps them with the struggles that they face in day to day life. It helps them to overcome things that they never thought they would be able to overcome. The following are just a few of the hundreds of benefits that meditation

can provide you with:

2. Reducing stress is one of the main reasons that people decide to turn to meditation. As we learned earlier in this book, when we experience stress, our bodies release cortisol, the stress hormone. This can affect our body negatively, especially if we are exposed to it long-term such as when we suffer from chronic anxiety or stress. We can suffer from depression, anxiety, high blood pressure, inability to think clearly, disrupted sleep, and fatigue all because of this one stress hormone. Studies have actually shown that when we meditate, the inflammation in our body is reduced. They have also shown that meditation helps to reduce stress and reduce symptoms of stress-related disorders such as post-traumatic stress disorder, IBS, and fibromyalgia.

3. Meditation helps us to control our anxiety. Of course, since meditation helps to reduce stress, we can assume that our anxiety levels are going to be less as well. However, what many people do not realize is that when they

meditate, they will see a reduction of symptoms of many different anxiety disorders such as social anxiety, OCD, phobias, and panic attacks. Many studies have been done, all showing that meditation helps to reduce anxiety and the symptoms of anxiety disorders. It has also been proven to help reduce job-related anxiety for those who work in high-pressure environments.

4. It helps to improve emotional health. Practicing meditation can help improve self-image and improve a person's outlook on life. It has been proven to decrease depression symptoms and improve mood as well. It promotes positive thinking, and the results last long term.

5. Meditation is a wonderful way to become more self-aware. Meditation is going to help you understand who you are, get to know yourself, and grow into the person that you want to be. It can help you overcome negative self-talk as well as self-defeating behaviors. It has been shown to help those who are suffering from chronic illness feel

more positive about what the future held for them. Studies have also shown that when those 60 and older practice meditation, they feel less lonely than those who did not.

6. When we meditate, we lengthen our attention span. This is great for those who are suffering from attention issues such as ADHD. Several studies have been done that have proven that those who practice meditation are able to stay focused on a task longer than those that do not meditate. They are also better able to remember details and important information. It can help to end worrying all of the time, increase attention, and reduce mind wandering. The good news is that you don't have to meditate for hours. In fact, meditating daily for just a short period of time is enough for you to start increasing your attention span.

7. Meditation improves memory, and it may reduce the chances of developing memory loss at a later age. When the mind is clear and focused, it stays young. It has been shown that those who practiced meditation at a

younger age were better able to care for themselves during their old age. Even those who have already developed dementia can benefit from meditation. It can actually help to improve their memory.

8. Meditation can make us kinder. Positive meditation is going to help increase the positivity in your life. It will change the way that you think about circumstances, how you relate to people, and how you look at life in general. You will think more positively about life, about yourself, and about other people. When you practice positive meditation, you are inviting positivity in your life and allowing yourself the ability to be kind to those around you, forgiving those who have hurt you, and helping those in need. On top of this, positive meditation can help improve social anxiety, anger management, and improve your marriage.

9. We have all heard about people getting hypnotized in order to overcome an addiction, but did you know that it is possible for you to use meditation to do the exact same thing?

Meditation helps people learn how to increase their willpower, redirect their attention, understand why they behave in certain ways, and control their emotions. Studies have even shown that meditation can help those suffering from alcoholism reduce their chance of relapse by helping them learn how to control their cravings. This can also be used when it comes to weight loss. Imagine how much weight you could lose if you could control your cravings.

10. Meditation improves sleep. Each night before I go to bed, I take the time to meditate. I know that if I do not do this, I am going to spend the night staring at the ceiling because I suffer from severe insomnia. However, when I meditate, I drift off to sleep in no time. Research has found that those who meditate fall asleep faster and are able to stay asleep longer than people who did not meditate. Meditation helps the body to relax, and it helps to relieve tension. This prepares your body for sleep and allows you to not worry about the struggles of the day.

11. Meditation can be used to help control pain. The way that we feel pain is connected to our state of mind. Have you ever met someone who had a really high pain tolerance? When we are in a stressful situation, our pain tolerance actually drops. One study looked at 3,500 people, and it found that when they meditated, they felt less pain associated with chronic diseases. It is suggested that meditation be part of treatment for those that have been diagnosed with terminal illnesses. Time and again, it has been shown that while two people can suffer from the same pain caused by the same thing when one person meditates, they experience less pain than the person that does not meditate.

12. Meditation can improve our physical health as well as our mental health, and one of the ways that it does this is by reducing blood pressure. When a person has high blood pressure, their heart has to work much harder than normal to pump blood to the rest of their body. As we already discussed, this can cause

the heart to function poorly, which can lead to a stroke or heart attack. Studies have shown that it is possible for our blood pressure to be reduced simply by spending time meditating each day. Wouldn't you like to get off of that blood pressure medication and actually start seeing real results? Meditation is able to reduce blood pressure levels because it turns off the fight or flight response in the body.

There are many different types of meditation, and you can meditate anywhere that you choose. You do not have to make a spectacle of yourself when you meditate, but instead, you can do it without anyone ever knowing. This is something that all of us can do in order to improve not only our emotional and mental health but our physical health as well. You do not have to have some special technique and can find plenty of guided meditations online for you to use until you feel comfortable meditating on your own.

Try out a few different styles of meditation and see which one you like the best. I do suggest that you give meditation a go for no less than 30 days. In 30 days, you will start seeing results if you are consistent with your meditation practices.

How to Meditate

Meditation is so simple, but it can be life-changing as well. It can improve your mental health, your emotional health, and your physical health. However, many people just don't do it. We all live these crazy busy lives where we are always on the go. We run from one place to another and barely have time to sit down and eat our meals, so how are we supposed to find time to meditate?

The good news is that meditation does not have to take a long time. You can meditate at any time during the day while you are working, on your lunch break, while you are exercising in the morning, or right before you go to bed.

There are so many ways to meditate that there is no way for me to cover them all; however, I am going to share with you a few techniques that I use.

The first technique that I use is called guided meditation. This is the easiest technique that I have found. All you have to do is put your earbuds in and listen. I found a guided meditation online that I enjoyed listening to, and I found it very relaxing.

There are many out there, and some of them are much more relaxing than others. I promise you that you will have to listen to more than one in order to find one that works for you because, as you can imagine, some of the voices that you will hear just are not that relaxing. For me, it is a man's voice talking calmly and deeply. That is what I find to be most relaxing.

This is the type of meditation that I use when I am working, like right now, when I am exercising, or when I am going to bed at night. It is perfectly okay if you fall asleep during meditation because your subconscious is still going to benefit. That is what is so great about guided meditation.

Anytime that I feel like I am struggling with a specific issue, such as productivity, or positivity, I will go and find a guided meditation that focuses on that one specific area of my life, and I will listen to it while I am working in order to get the most out of my time. Not only do I start seeing improvements right away, but I see them for a very long time.

Meditating without being guided is also something that I do. I do this in the car (of course, with my eyes open) or when I am out and about doing my errands.

I also do this when I need something a little extra to get me through.

The first thing that you will want to do is choose a place. Sometimes I like to go off by myself and just meditate. I don't want to hear any noise, but instead, I want peace and just spend time with myself. You can sit down, or stand, or continue doing whatever task it is that you are doing. Just make sure that you are not slouching. Good posture is important to our health.

Close your eyes if possible, keep them open if you are driving or doing anything except for sitting or lying down. Relax every muscle in your body, starting at your toes and working your way all the way up to the top of your head. Inhale through your nose and out your mouth as you relax each of these muscles.

Become aware of how your body is feeling. Really feel those muscles loosening up and become mindful of the moment. Don't worry about all of the chaos that is going on around you. Don't worry about the bills that need to be paid or the project that is due tomorrow morning. Focus on right now. If you find that your thoughts are straying to other things, just bring them back and feel your body relaxing.

Once you feel completely relaxed, you can open

your eyes (or not if they were already opened) and continue on with your day. If you decided to take some time to yourself, stand up and stretch, allowing the blood to flow to every part of your body before you go and focus on your next activity. That really is all there is to it.

Some people may find that it is easier for them to meditate if they have some sort of relaxing music going on in the background, and this is perfectly fine. In fact, listening to relaxing music while you meditate is a great idea because when you hear that particular music in the future, your body is going to know that it is time to meditate.

Q&A

1. How often do I meditate?

Many people find themselves wondering how often they should meditate. Is this a once a week thing that we do? Not really. You should make sure that you are meditating at least once per day. I prefer a little bit more. Even when I am busy and don't have a lot of time during the day, I make sure that I meditate in the morning as well as when I am going to bed.

This may seem like just one more thing to do when

you first start out, just one more chore to add to the list, but as you learn how to meditate, you are going to start enjoying it. You are going to start seeing it as something that you look forward to each day and not just something else that has to be done.

2. How long should I meditate?

When you first start out, you should try to get in at least 15 minutes per mediation session. Most of the time, your mind is not even going to settle down for at least 10 minutes. This means that if you only meditate for 10 minutes, you really are not going to see the benefits. If later, you find that you want to meditate longer, that is totally fine. I know of people who meditate for two hours in the morning. While this is not something even I would aim to do (I like to sleep far too much), it is achievable.

3. I find it very hard to sit still and concentrate while meditating.

Many people struggle with this but remember what I said at the beginning of the chapter. Mediation is not about focusing, sitting still, or concentrating on one thing. That is more along the lines of visualization. If you need to be up moving around while you meditate, that is perfectly fine. If you want to meditate while you are exercising or while you are working, that is fine as well. You need to focus on doing what works best for you and don't worry about what other people think. You see, the way that I meditate is not going to be the way that you meditate, and that is not going to be the way that someone else meditates. We all do it our own way, and you just have to figure out what way that is.

4. I am afraid that if I meditate, I will be going against my religious beliefs. What can I do?

Meditation is not a religion, and it does not go against any religion. You have to remember that you are not praying to a deity. You are not praying to anyone. You do not have to focus on any religious texts or icons. If you come across a guided meditation that asks you to do something like this, just move on to the next one.

5. I keep falling asleep when I am meditating, what can I do?

As I already mentioned, if you are practicing guided meditation, then it is okay for you to fall asleep while you are meditating. Your subconscious is still going to benefit. If you are meditating on your own and falling asleep, that is okay as well. This just shows that your body is in a completely relaxed state. On the other hand, if you are in a situation where you don't want to fall asleep, such as at your desk, at work, you will want to take a few steps to reduce the chances of that from happening. First of all, you will want to make sure that you are letting in enough light. If you are meditating with your eyes closed, open them. If this does not work, I suggest meditating just before bed instead of when you are out of the house or at work.

How Does Meditation Affect the Vagus Nerve?

Meditation and the vagus nerve are very important to one another. They both work together, and they both need each other in order to work properly. You have probably already noticed that meditation can have many of the same effects on the body as stimulating the vagus nerve. It is believed that this is because the benefits of meditation are caused by stimulating the vagus nerve.

Mindful meditation, which is when we focus on being fully present at the moment that is happening right now, seems to be the most effective meditation to stimulate the vagus nerve. Mindful meditation seems to be the most effective because it helps us to be present at this exact moment. We are no longer focusing on what has happened in the past, nor what may happen in the future. We experience each moment fully.

Mindfulness can enhance all other forms of meditation as well, which can increase the benefits significantly. If you practice meditation, you do not have to practice any of the other methods for stimulating your vagus nerve; however, if you do, it is only going to cause your results to be concentrated.

When we meditate, our brain sends a message to our nervous system, which tells the body to stop the fight or flight response. This is necessary if we want to stimulate the vagus nerve and reduce the stress, depression, anxiety, pain, or other issues that we are facing.

By practicing meditation, we are able to take control of the functions of our bodies that were once through to be automatic. This is very important because not only does it show us that we can literally heal our bodies through stimulating the vagus nerve through meditation, but it allows us to understand that our own health and wellbeing is ours to control.

CHAPTER 16
YOGA TREATMENTS FOR VAGUS NERVE

Vagus nerve stimulation therapy can eliminate drug cravings

Dependence on any substance can make the life of an individual upside down. From spending a fortune to deluding own family, an individual dependent on unlawful substances can go to any degree. Be that as it may, how does fixation power somebody to put such a great amount in question and after that lose all? There are a few variables having an effect on everything with regards to managing the developing issue of addiction.

Desires are a major issue that torment various individuals battling drug fixation, particularly when they attempt to fall off the addictive substance. Incidentally, numerous individuals would have effectively accomplished long haul moderation if yearnings didn't manifest with fixation. Aside from being considered as the significant deterrents in recuperation treatment, longings are likewise the main driver of backsliding.

A total recuperation from habit happens just when an individual is free from longings. Carrying on with a sans drug existence without the requirement for steady checking against drug longings can be hard for a recouping individual; however, an ongoing report distributed in the diary Learning and Memory has recommended that drug yearnings can be viably treated with vagus nerve stimulation (VNS) therapy. Under the therapy, the patients are shown new practices that supplant their old addictive conduct of looking for drugs.

Job Of VNS In Habit Recuperation

In the University of Texas at Dallas study, the scientists uncovered that the VNS therapy helped patients to recuperate from the maladaptive conduct of drug-taking. VNS is fundamentally a careful procedure wherein a gadget is embedded to a wire strung along the vagus nerve, which goes up from the neck to the brain and interfaces with the zone responsible for directing state of mind. Measured as little as a silver dollar, the gadget works simply like a pacemaker.

The strategy is endorsed by the U.S. Nourishment and Drug Administration (FDA) and is considered as a potential treatment for treatment-safe depression, post-traumatic stress disorder (PTSD), and loss of motion. The investigation further featured that VNS encourages "termination learning" of drug-chasing practices by decreasing desires and supplanting the conduct related to compulsion with new ones. "Annihilation of frightful recollections and termination of drug-chasing recollections depends on a similar substrate in the brain. In our trials, VNS encourages both the termination learning and diminishes the backslide response also," said Dr. Sven Kroener of the University of Texas at Dallas.

Sans Drug Life Is Conceivable

In spite of the fact that addictive substances prevail in incidentally mitigating emotional and physical torments of drug abusers, they need to, in the long run, adapt to the agonizing indications of substance misuse. Other than building up various physical and mental issues, a considerable lot of these people additionally become foolish and self-destructive in nature.

Dependence on any substance can be dangerous. Just a far-reaching treatment program, including detoxification, medications, psychotherapies, and other experiential treatments like yoga, meditation, and so forth, can enable a person to get calm. Additionally, an all-encompassing recuperation of the executives' plan is similarly essential to continue the time of restraint and oversee longings. In any case, the degree to which medicinal services professionals can accumulate brings about the treatment for drug dependence is subject to the clinical qualities of the patients that may shift as indicated by the sort of drug being manhandled just as its quantity, term and the strategy for utilizing the drug (oral or intravenous).

CHAPTER 17
EXERCISES TO BALANCE THE VAGUS NERVE

When your Vagus nerve is healthy, it supports all sorts of parts of your body, including helping you sleep better, deeply relax, and even bounce back from injury faster. But how do you make sure this nerve stays healthy and properly functioning? Thankfully you can learn how to regulate this nerve on your own without the intervention of a medical professional, in most cases. When you know how to regulate and heal your Vagus nerve, you can help reduce chronic inflammation, help you overcome migraines, reduce symptoms of chronic auto-immune disease, depression, and anxiety.

There is a scenario where you may no longer be able to sense when something or someone is safe or not accurately. This happens when you are chronically exposed to trauma for a long time. This means you could be in a safe situation but respond as if being threatened. You react by fighting, freezing, running away, or fainting. But over time and practice, you can learn how to "override" these responses to support a healthy response to a non-threatening situation. If you have a disorder affecting or originating from your Vagus nerve, you can learn ways to stimulate your social engagement system. The more you practice this, the stronger the myelinated Vagus nerve pathway becomes. The more you activate this, the fattier coating in the myelinated Vagal nerve, helping increase both control and speed of information sharing.

You can safely mobilize and immobilize your Vagus nerve using mind and body therapies that you can do at home. These therapies allow you to regulate the Vagus nerve and enhance your resilience. To be able to create this capacity, you first need to create the ability to feel connected, calm, and at peace. Being able to do this is the foundation. Then you can build upon it by tapping into your social engagement system and construct your tolerance for activation during distressing physiological situations. To achieve this, you need to learn how to combine your social engagement system with both immobilization and mobilization, leading to a re-establishment of the sense of security while operating in those states of your nervous system.

Somatic psychology and the therapies for your mind and body require you to observe and engage in different present-moment situations, such as your thoughts, emotional experiences, breath, and the sensations in the body. These methodologies also assist you in observing and acknowledging your external environment, reaffirming that you are indeed safe in the present moment. Using physical movement is one form of these therapies, like walking meditations, tai chi, and yoga. Other therapies use complete stillness to help with this process. These include things like yoga Nidra, relaxation techniques, and supine or seated meditation.

An Example Practice for Healing Your Vagus Nerve

You can practice different engagement and stimulation of your Vagus nerve, using methods that require stillness and then others that require movement, so you practice blending social engagement for different energy and health requirements. The following example is designed to help your health and support your Vagus nerve.

- Select a safe location. Identify and locate yourself in a non-threatening environment to begin your practice. When there, find a comfortable place to lie down, sit, or stand. You will need to be in this position for a few minutes, so take a moment to choose a position that supports your comfort. When in position, look around you and find "clues" that tell you that you are in a safe space. After finding a few cues, repeat to yourself quietly, "I am safe right now. I am connected to this world. I am peaceful."

- Enhance your awareness of your senses. Begin deepening your breath, focusing on long and slow inhales and exhales. Pay attention to how breathing through your nose feels. Identify the subtle movements in your body with each breath. Shift your focus to the sound of your breath. Take a few breaths just listening to the sounds of your inhales and the sounds of your exhale. And now shift your focus again, this time to your awareness of other sensations in your body. Repeat the saying from step one to yourself in your mind, "I am safe right now. I am connected to this world. I am peaceful." If you feel anxiety or any other mental or physical distress, return to step one, looking around you to find the clues that tell your body that you are safe.

- Experiment with mindfully mobilizing your Vagus nerve. Try by increasing your breathing rate. Move your body. This can include getting into an active yoga posture or walk-in in swiftly. You can also dance to music. Move just enough to increase your heart rate and quicken your breath to support you as you move. Repeat the saying again, "I am safe right now. I am connected to this world. I am peaceful." Again, if you are feeling distressed or anxious, return to step one and visually orient yourself back into your safe space.

- Experiment with mindful immobilization of your Vagus nerve. Now it is time to bring your body back to stillness, whether that is returning to the comfortable position you began in, or by lying down, sitting, or standing still. Encourage your body to be as still as possible and witness your heart rate slowing down. Let your body press firmly into the ground, letting the Earth or the floor hold you. Bring your attention back to breathing deeply and slowly. If you feel comfortable, try extending yours exhales to be even longer than your inhales. This helps stimulate the feeling of relaxation. If you are tightening or tensing any muscles, relax them now. Say to yourself quietly, "I am safe right now. I am connected to this world. I am peaceful." If you find yourself anxious or distressed, return to step one to remind yourself that you are in a safe place.

25 Additional Self-guided Healing Exercises

- **Cold temperatures:** studies have indicated that when your body has to adjust to colder temperatures, it increases your parasympathetic response system to allow you to relax, thereby inhibiting your sympathetic response. This process is overseen by your Vagus nerve. And this does not need to be extreme exposure to cold; just a small amount of cold exposure can activate your Vagus nerve. One method you can try is dipping your face in ice-cold water or taking a cold shower. You can also expose yourself to cold by going outside in cold temperatures or standing in front of the open freezer door. Drinking ice-cold water is also effective.

- **Chant or sing.** You can easily increase the variability in your heart rate when you sing. You can change this variability in different ways when you sing energetically, sing hymns, chant mantras, or hum. The reason this is effective is because of the stimulation of the vagal pump on your throat. If you sing at the top of your lungs, you can engage the back muscles in your throat, activating your Vagus nerve. It also triggers your sympathetic nervous system along with your Vagus nerve. Also, singing is shown to increase oxytocin production.

- **Practice yoga.** Yoga is generally beneficial in increasing activity in the parasympathetic system and activation of your Vagus nerve. In one study, participants were either assigned a walking process to help them stabilize their mood and lower anxiety while another group participated in yoga. Those that participated in yoga had increased levels of thalamic GABA, which was associated with their improved mood, mood stability, and lowered anxiety levels.

- **Practice meditation.** Two different "methods" for meditation have been shown to help activate the Vagus nerve, chanting "om" and "loving-kindness" guided meditation. Chanting "om" is related to the benefits of singing. "Loving kindness" guided meditation assists in people visualizing a positive and peaceful state. The success of these meditation methods is shown in the measurement of heart rate variability before, during, and after meditation.

- **Engaging in positive relationships in social settings.** In a study, participants were instructed to meditate. One group was given the mantra to repeat to themselves, "May you feel safe, may you feel happy, may you be healthy, may you live with ease" while visualizing others in a compassionate manner. The other group was given meditation instructions that did not foster a compassionate connection to others. Those that had kind thoughts about other people increased their positive emotions, like hope, peace, amusement, interest, joy, and love. The presence of these increased emotions also correlated with an increase in heart rate variability and a stimulated Vagus nerve.

- **Practice deep and slow breathing techniques.** Just taking a few deep breaths can calm you down by stimulating your Vagus nerve. Baroreceptors are in your neck and transmit messages to your brain when your heart rate and blood pressure are too low or too high. When you practice slow and deep breathing, you can increase the sensitivity of their receptors and also activate your Vagus nerve. This, in turn, lowers anxiety and blood pressure. An average adult that takes about six breaths in a minute will promote rest and relaxation. As you breathe, focus on ballooning your stomach out as you inhale, letting the oxygen reach into the lower lobes of your lungs, and as you exhale, pull your navel in to cave in your stomach, pressing out all the oxygen from the lower parts of your lungs. The more dramatic the ballooning and sinking of your stomach, the deeper your breath is on average.

- **Laugh a lot**. The more you laugh, the more you stimulate your Vagus nerve and calm your body. Studies have shown many times that this really is one of the "best medicines." There are reports where people fainted from laughing too much. This is likely due to the overstimulation of the Vagus nerve and the parasympathetic nervous system. The sensation becomes extreme and activates the immobilization response. In addition, people that experience this response to laughter often have an illness called Angelman's, which is a fairly rare condition. It is connected to the overstimulation of the Vagus nerve. Also, activation of the Vagus nerve can result in laughter. There are many benefits to laughter in addition to stimulating the Vagus nerve, including lowering the risk of heart disease, improving cognitive functioning, and increasing beta-endorphins.

- **Pray often to your divine source or spiritual guide**. Praying to a higher power has shown to activate the Vagus nerve. The studies conducted where on Catholics reciting the rosary prayer in particular; however, it is likely that any prayer to a divine connection can most likely stimulate your Vagus nerve in a similar function. Researchers found that prayer enhanced the rhythm of the heart, improving the resting heart rate as well as the heart rate variability. One observation unique to the study on this reciting the rosary prayer was that the prayer took ten seconds to recite, meaning the participants had to take a breath that lasted for ten seconds, resulting in an average of about six breaths per minute. If you recall earlier, it was explained in the section about breathing exercises that breathing at this slow rate is good for activating your Vagus nerve. It increases your heart rate variability, thereby activating your Vagus nerve.

- **Use PEMF or magnetic field stimulation.** This is something similar to what patients are given to activate a Vagus nerve stimulator that was surgically placed in the body but does not require the surgical intervention in your body. These small devices send pulses into your body to stimulate the Vagus nerve. You can use them on your digestive tract, neck, and skull. It can help in reducing inflammation, regulate digestion, and improved relaxation.

1. **Eat probiotics regularly.** The gut is connected to the brain by the Vagus nerve. When your gut is "out of order," it affects your brain. So, when you take care of your digestive tract and stomach, you can improve the communication process of the Vagus nerve, and thereby improving the communication of other organs with the brain as well. A study conducted on animals being given a probiotic called Lactobacillus Rhamnosus showed a positive alteration to their GABA levels. These levels are handled by the Vagus nerve.

2. **Get in more and better exercise for your body.** You do not need to do cross-fit or become a bodybuilder to activate and regulate your Vagus nerve. Just a mild form of exercise can help stimulate your digestion. Digestion is

regulated by the Vagus nerve. This means that when you exercise, you are stimulating and activating your Vagus nerve, supporting healthy gut function.

3. **Get a massage.** There are certain areas on your body that connect to your Vagus nerve more superficially. This means that you can access this Vagus nerve easier from the outside of your body. The carotid sinus, tucked in your neck, is known to help stimulate your Vagus nerve. It is easily accessible during a massage. It is known to help prevent and reduce seizures in patients. Using mild and firm pressure during a massage can help stimulate the Vagus nerve. Infant massage is common therapy parents and caregivers can use to help a baby gain weight. The process stimulates the digestive process, which is regulated and controlled by the Vagus nerve. When the Vagus nerve is stimulated and activated, particularly in the abdominal region, digestion can be improved. Also, massaging your feet can help improve heart rate variability and improve the function of the

Vagus nerve. It lowers your heart rate and your blood pressure. All of these benefits are known to lower the risk of developing heart disease.

4. **Participate in regular intermittent fasting.** This is an old healing therapy used to help heal many illnesses. Intermittent fasting or reduction in caloric intake can increase your heart rate variability and stimulate your Vagus nerve. There are many studies that show the health benefits of fasting and your well-being. Your metabolism decreases during a fast, which is regulated by your Vagus nerve. Also, your Vagus nerve observes when your blood glucose lowers, and your gut's stimuli decrease both chemically and mechanically. Your metabolic rate lowers while your Vagus nerve increases, all because of the impulses transmitted to the brain from your liver. While fasting, there is also a decrease in your CRH and CCK, with an increase in NPY, all of which are hormones. But when you eat, everything is flip-flopped. When food is introduced, the signals from your gut increase your

sympathetic response. This leads to more stressor responses, such as higher levels of CCK and CRH, and lower levels of NPY. In animal studies, some patients showed that fasting could improve the subdiaphragmatic Vagus nerve activity. Also, fasting increased estrogen receptors in parts of the brain, making you more receptive and sensitive to estrogen, also a link to the Vagus nerve activation.

5. **Rest on your right-hand side.** There are a few studies that indicate laying or sleeping on your right side helps increase your heart rate variability and activates your Vagus nerve. This is the best side to lay on, while the next best is to lie on your left side. Lying on your back leads to the lowest activation of your Vagus nerve. Resting on this side is directly related to your heart, but also applies appropriate pressure and support of your Vagal response.

6. **Gargle liquids**. When you activate the back of your throat, you activate your Vagus nerve. This is because the muscles in the back of your

throat must contract and release to engage, such as when gargling. This contraction in the back of the throat and these muscles mean the Vagus nerve is activated. It also stimulates your digestive tract. You do not need to gargle just mouthwash. You can also practice gargling water any time you take a sip of water before swallowing so that you are constantly engaging, contracting, and activating your Vagus nerves, digestion, and mouth muscles.

7. **Eat more seafood to increase DHA and EPA in your diet.** DHA and EPA are known to lower your heart rate and also increase your heart rate variability. These two "side effects" of these nutrients are evidence that they stimulate your Vagus nerve. The amount of these two nutrients is still uncertain, and more studies are needed to directly correlate the Vagus nerve to the intake of DHA and EPA from seafood, but early evidence suggests it is connected. There are plenty of studies that show the health benefits of these nutrients in other aspects, as well as why eating seafood

is a good diet decision. Regardless of the lack of scientific evidence for this self-guided exercise, it is still a good health decision.

8. **Stimulate the release of oxytocin.** When your body releases oxytocin, it helps lower your appetite as well as increase relaxation. The levels of this hormone increase when the Vagus nerve is active, sending messages from the digestive tract to the brain. In one study on mice that had their Vagus nerve removed showed that even though the oxytocin was still released, it did not have the same effect on the subjects. For example, the mice without Vagus nerves did not have lowered appetites compared to mice who had a fully functioning Vagus nerve.

9. **Increase the amount of zinc you consume.** Zinc is a common mineral in foods and in supplements, but surprisingly many humans do not consume enough. In a study where rats were given a diet low or deficient in zinc for three days, it was clear the Vagus nerve was not functioning at full capacity. When zinc was reintroduced, the Vagus nerve

was activated and stimulated.

10. **Use a tongue depressor**. This self-guided exercise may sound "hoaky" at first, but think about when you are at the doctor, and they use a tongue depressor to check the back of your throat. Do you often gag when they do this? Remember, gagging activates your Vagus nerve! If you are uncertain how to make yourself gag, this is the answer. Combine gagging with singing, and you are effectively "working out" your Vagus nerve, giving it plenty of different stimulation and activation.

11. **See an acupuncturist.** This is not typically something you can do to yourself, but it is something that can make a large difference in the stimulation and function of your Vagus nerve. Thousands of years ago, before they called it the Vagus nerve, practitioners recognized that there are certain points on the body that stimulate this nerve and that you can access this from small intrusions into the body with needles. One of the most traditional locations for stimulating

the Vagus nerve is on the ear. One famous "case" of acupuncture and Vagus nerve stimulation is the death of a man whose heart rate lowered too low during the session.

12.   **Chew gum.** It is like turning on the lights when you chew gum or complete the action known as CCK. Chewing gum or another substance in a similar manner for an extended period of time allows you to reduce the amount of food you eat in one sitting. This is a reduction in appetite. Your appetite is controlled in part by your Vagus nerve. The Vagus nerve is responsible for sending information from your stomach and digestive tract about your hunger, but CCK reduces this. This is evidence that the Vagus nerve is activated to reduce this craving.

13.   **Eat a more fibrous diet.** If you want to feel fuller and slow down your stomach emptying its contents into your small intestine, you want the Vagus nerve to tell the brain that it is satisfied while eating earlier in the process. To do this, you should increase GLP-1 hormone levels. One of the best ways

to do this is to eat more fiber.

14. **Give yourself or get a coffee enema.** Your Vagus nerve essentially ends in your digestive tract. It plays a large role here and is also easily impacted here. If you are able to increase your bowel, you can increase your activation of the Vagus nerve. One method for increasing your bowel is with an enema.

15. **Cough or engage your abdominal muscles.** Think about how you feel after having a bowel movement. Most likely, your body is more relaxed, and you feel "better." The process of having a bowel movement requires you to engage certain muscles with intense and strong activation. This engagement of these muscles helps stimulate your Vagus nerve.

16. **Get out in the sunshine.** It may sound counter-intuitive given what we know about the harmful rays of the sun and our skin; however, the sun is a good source of MSH or Alpha-MSH. In studies on rats, an introduction of Alpha-MSH helped lower the risk of stroke because of the lowering of inflammation and

the activation of the Vagus nerve. In another study, subjects were injected with Alpha-MSH directly into the brain with results showing moderate activation of the Vagus nerve for some subjects with various conditions. While you cannot inject yourself in the brain with this, you can sit outside in the sun and let your skin absorb this nutrient for you, engaging your Vagus nerve.

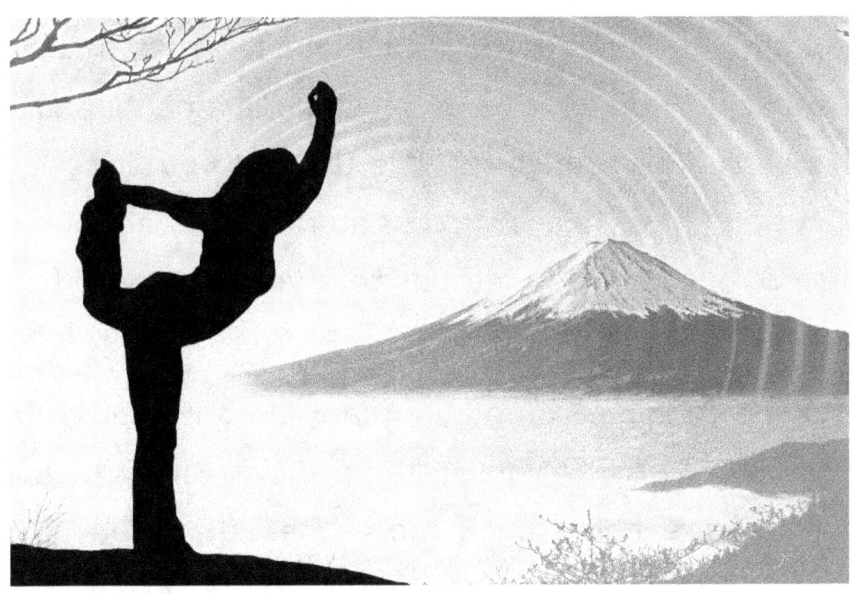

CHAPTER 18
ACTIVATING YOUR VAGUS NERVE EFFORTLESSLY

While everyone is born with different levels of vagal tone, you can have an effect on it. If your vagal tone is low, there are steps you can take to activate your vagus nerve and improve its tone. I have personally tried a large number of the activities and techniques mentioned in this book. The remainder, I've talked to other people about and have heard success stories for every one of them. These are all methods that you can try to help boost your vagal tone.

Some of these you may already do but need to be more conscious as you do them. Some are new and may require being a bit more open than you have been in the past. For example, if you're not used to acupressure or meditation, these can seem odd and out of place. The great thing about this is that you can pick and choose what you want to try. If one activity isn't the right fit for you, make sure to replace it with something else.

Most people are looking for easy fixes, and while there is no complete cure that doesn't require a little work, you can certainly implement the following methods into your daily life without much effort at all.

Positive Relationships

Your relationships have quite an effect on every aspect of your life, from health and mood to your self-confidence. It's best to surround yourself with positive relationships and people who lift you up. Doing this will not only make you feel happier, but it will also increase your vagus nerve tone and build your immune system.

The vagus nerve is responsible for oxytocin release, the hormone that is essential in human and animal bonding. It makes sense then that it can all affect you when speaking with someone else. If you are talking to someone who is negative or frightens you, then your stress response is activated, your heart rate goes up, and other unpleasant effects occur.

It has also been proven in studies that people who have a higher tone in their vagus nerve tend to be kinder and to bond better with others. If this isn't enough reason to be social, then you might want to look into making more human contact to find out what it feels like. However, this can also be activated when you are around animals. They love unconditionally and can make sure you get lots of positivity.

Regular interaction with other people can lift your spirits an amazing amount. It's easy these days to focus on just being online, but it doesn't count. The technology, while it allows us to communicate, doesn't allow for the person to person interaction that our brains and bodies require.

Getting a genuine hug from someone can tone your vagus nerve. If you get several hugs every day, you'll find that your mood improves. Both eye contact and human touch have massive effects on how toned your vagus nerve is. Every time you spend time with someone else, whether it's laughing over a cup of coffee or holding hands as you walk down the street, your vagus nerve is being stimulated.

Human connection can help you feel calmer, more positive, and improves your mood overall. The effects can last for days, in some situations.

Security and Self-Love

When you feel safe, your vagal tone improves. The same goes for feeling happy and positive.

Unfortunately, most people don't really like themselves or their bodies. They find it difficult to take a compliment and will put themselves down. They feel guilty and unhappy about things and are often stressed out, feeling that they just aren't good enough.

Feeling positive about your body and loving who you are can also improve your vagal tone. Self-love is one of the biggest changes you can make in your life, with positive results in your health. You'll find that your immune system functions more efficiently when you are happy with yourself.

Security is another big part of being in control of your life and improving vagal tone. If you feel unsafe, you deal with stress and anxiety. It isn't necessary to have a physical threat right there, though. You can feel stressed if you aren't feeling safe in general. And in today's world, it's very difficult to feel safe. There's always something to worry about.

This was one of the more significant issues that I faced after my vagus nerve was damaged. Before the antibiotic ruined my body, I rarely felt anxious or stressed. All that changed after my vagus nerve was damaged. Suddenly, I was dealing with far more anxiety than before. In addition to the pain, I felt panicky every time I had to do anything outside my comfort zone. Then it got worse. I ended up anxious and stressed over the simplest of things. Even picking my children up from school became a difficult situation. My brain raced over all the things that could go wrong at any given moment, and I never truly felt safe.

How can you increase your feeling of security? That depends on the person. In some cases, you may need to take physical steps to make yourself feel safer. This could mean you take the time to install locks on your doors, get a guard dog, etc. These will help you feel safer on the outside. However, you also need to feel secure mentally.

Create a space for yourself where you can relax and detox from the stress of everyday life. This should be an area that reduces anxiety and makes you feel happy and loved. Feeling secure can help your vagus nerve increase tone, so it's worth working on this.

Having a high vagal tone also helps with feeling safe, so it's a cycle that only strengthens as you improve it.

Gratitude

Don't underestimate the power of positive thinking on your vagus nerve health. In fact, it has been proven that a grateful attitude is most prevalent in those with high vagal tone. If your vagal tone is high when you're resting, you are more likely to experience pleasant feelings like gratitude, compassion, love, and will be happier than those with low vagal tone.

You can build on this happiness and increase your vagus nerve tone by developing a habit of being grateful. This is like any other habit, where you need to keep building on it regularly. Here are a few ways you can increase your gratitude:

Keep a gratitude journal: Make a point of writing down at least three things every day that you're grateful for. There will be days when you don't feel like anything is worth saying thanks for, but there is always something. It may be a little thing, like being able to get up in the morning or coffee. There's no shortage of things that you can be thankful for. By focusing on these things every single day, you'll eventually start noticing more things to be grateful for, and this will only build.

Say thank you every day: People do things for you every day. Even if they are supposed to do it because it's their job, such as a waitress or bank teller, be sure to say thank you. That little bit of gratitude can have a bit impact, not only on your life but on other people's lives. You can even go a bit further if you want by leaving a generous tip or even a note.

Be with people you love: You can't help but feel grateful and happy when you are around those you love. Make a point of spending time with those special people. Have some tea together, go for a walk, or just sit and chat. You'll find yourself calmer and happier when you spend time with these people.

Be mindful: It's easy to start going through your day on rote, not really thinking about what you're doing as you do the same things you do every day. It's important to stay present as you complete your daily tasks. You can do this by focusing on what you are doing and finding pleasure in the individual task that you are accomplishing. Even doing the dishes can be an enlightening experience if you focus.

Choose happiness: It's important to decide to be happy. This doesn't always work, of course, because you can feel other emotions, and sometimes, they are more than overwhelming. However, happiness is often a choice, and you need to make that choice every day. When you wake up in the morning, take a moment to think about your life and decide that today, you will be happy.

Your daily attitude will have a lot to do with vagal tone. It's also beneficial to your mental attitude to be happy and calm. If it takes raising your vagal tone to do that, then you can start with the exercises I've shared here to get you started.

Diet and Eating Habits

You can improve many aspects of your health simply by eating correctly, but did you know that this also has a massive effect on your vagus nerve? I didn't realize until after I had already changed my eating habits that there were some other benefits to this lifestyle, including boosting vagal tone.

It turns out that what you eat and the bacteria in your digestive tract actually affect how your brain functions. The bacteria in your gut can get upset or become imbalanced when you take antibiotics or other types of medicines. That's exactly what happened to me. So when my friend told me to take probiotics, she was actually on the right track. It just takes more than a few bottles of kombucha to fix the gut.

What Foods Should You Eat?

The types of foods you eat are very important, but some are more so. Here are some foods that should be included in your daily diet:

Fermented Food: Fermented foods include healthy microbes and bacteria, so they can help restore your digestive tract bacteria if it has been depleted. Things like sauerkraut, cheese, kefir, kombucha, and yogurt are some of the more common fermented foods. However, you can also make fermented salsa, ketchup, and many other delicious, gut-boosting foods at home.

Foods High in Fiber: You want to keep things moving, and one of the signs that your gut is not healthy is constipation. It makes sense than to eat fiber, but there's another good reason for this . . . prebiotics. Your high fiber foods contain prebiotics that will help good gut bacteria flourish and reduce your stress levels. High fiber foods include anything made with whole grains, seeds, fruits and vegetables, and nuts.

Calcium: Known as the bone-building mineral, calcium helps protect the body against diseases like diabetes and cancer. It's also an essential part of keeping your nervous system and cardiovascular system functioning properly, which includes your vagus nerve. Calcium is one of the nutrients that the body cannot produce, so you need to eat it. You'll find calcium in dairy products, dark green leafy vegetables like kale or broccoli, and in canned fish with softened bones.

Magnesium: Without magnesium, the heart cannot function as well as it should. In fact, this mineral is an essential part of regulating the circulatory system. It helps the heart contract correctly, manages heart rhythm, and prevents many cardiac issues. It can be found in nuts and seeds, green leafy vegetables like kale and spinach, figs, avocado, bananas, and seafood in general. Legumes such as beans and peas are also rich in magnesium.

Sodium: Chances are you've heard that salt is bad for you all your life. It's a common misconception and, while too much sodium isn't great for the body, it is necessary for your body to function. Whole grain bread, cured meats, and chicken are all excellent sources of sodium. You can also use sea salt or Himalayan salt in your food.

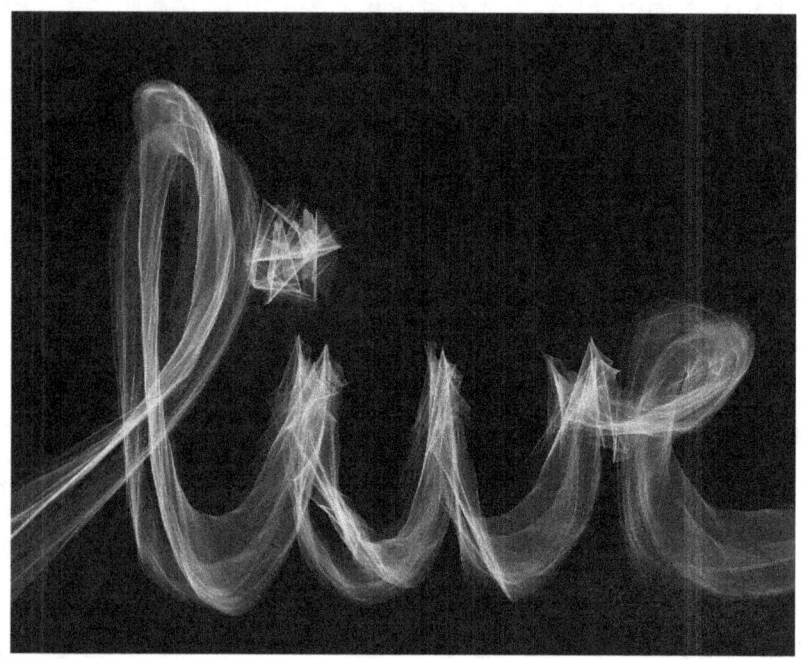

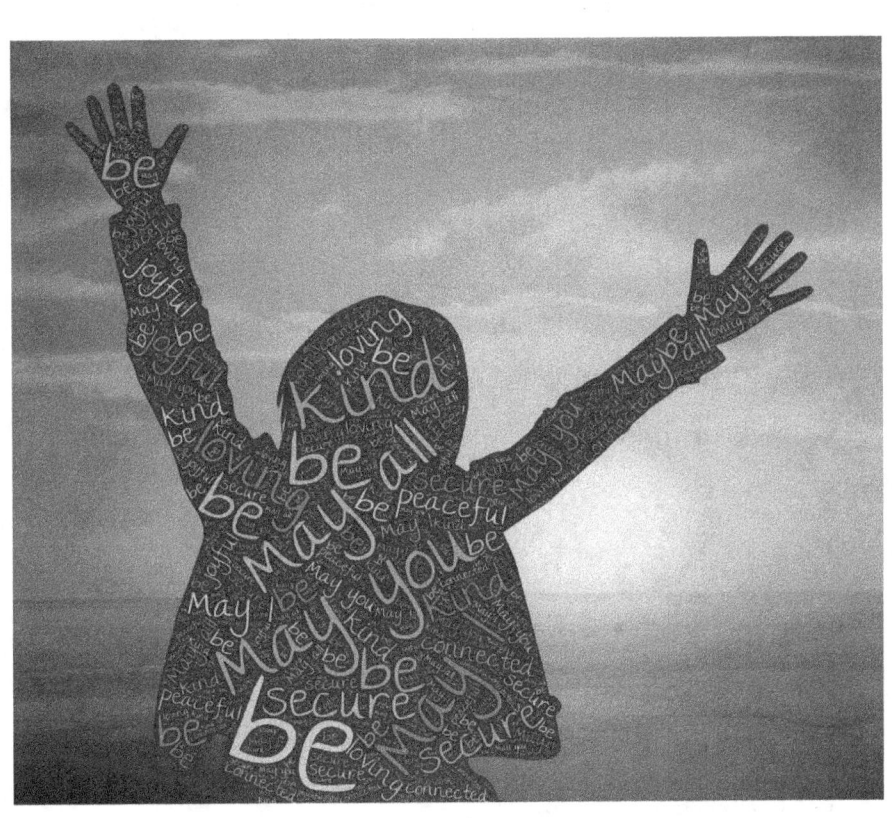

CHAPTER 19
MORE ACTIVITIES AND EXERCISES TO TRIGGER YOUR VAGUS NERVE

Even if exercise or any of the other previously mentioned methods of stimulating the vagus nerve aren't your things, that's okay. There are plenty of ways to get things moving and to activate your nervous system. You should also consider how much you need and how often to stimulate your nerves.

The following methods are a little more sedate and are easily done wherever you are. There's no need for special equipment, and all can be done quickly if you're pressed for time. In fact, you can turn your regular activities into vagal toning activities with a few small changes.

Music and Binaural Beats

Certain types of sound can help your brain work better. This has been known for a while now, but there are more and more studies being done on neuroplasticity and music. You may notice that music affects you. It can give you energy or make you feel low-key. Some music is anger-inducing, while other music can calm you. This is all very important to notice since you can actually make use of the noise to help your vagal tone.

Many people use music as a way to control their moods, but you can take it a step further and add in binaural beats. These are designed to stimulate the brain, but they are also used to tone the vagus nerve.

Binaural beats are two or more similar sine waves. They need to be pure tone and usually work best with earphones, as they are presented in each ear. As an example, a 500 Hz pure tone could be played in one ear, while a 480 Hz pure tone would be in the other ear. The result is an auditory illusion, which increases the neuroplasticity of the brain and makes it more open to memories and studying.

Binaural beats are considered entrainment, where a duo of autonomous rhythmic oscillators work together to interact and synchronize. This technology can be used to affect the body in various ways, including changing your heart rate, relaxation, and blood pressure, among other things. It is also used to boost memory and increase focus.

Regular music is often mixed with binaural beats to make it easier to listen to the odd rhythms. You can listen to the music while the binaural beats work with your brain to stimulate it and to create a higher state of alertness or a more relaxed state. Different beats are used, depending on the desired result. You can use them to help you sleep, to keep you awake without caffeine, and even to help regulate your moods and offset depression. They all work with the vagus nerve, so when used in conjunction with the other methods in this book, you'll find entrainment to be particularly effective in building vagal tone.

Even if you don't incorporate binaural beats into your vagal tone routine, you should definitely consider some music. Opt for something that you enjoy, and that feels good. You can listen to music on your morning commute to improve your mood and boost tone or use it whenever you have a short break.

Deep Breathing

When you're feeling stressed or anxious, you probably take a deep breath and let it out slowly. This is a natural way to slow your heart rate and reduce the fight or flight response. However, just one or two breaths is not enough to really tone your vagus nerve.

If you want to experience the long-term benefits of this, you should consider doing breathing exercises on a daily basis.

Deep breathing requires breathing from the diaphragm. As you inhale, your belly will expand. Aim to breathe in slowly and out just as slowly, taking about 5 seconds for each inhale and exhale. You should take roughly six breaths per minute. The normal rate is 12-15 breaths each minute, so this is slowing it down considerably.

This type of deep breathing will stimulate your vagus nerve and promote calmness. Try for 10-12 breaths to really bring your stress levels under control. Doing this daily will help build vagal tone and ward off undue stress in the future. It's also helpful to breathe like this whenever you find that you are getting anxious or feeling off. Deep breathing will slow your heart rate and help you calm down.

As you breathe, focus on the way your body pulls in the air. Imagine the oxygen moving into the blood and then being carried throughout your body. Feel the exhale and consciously deflate your body as you breathe out. It's all part of feeling more connected with your body and with your life, which also stimulates the vagus nerve and helps build its tone.

Meditation

Did you know you can affect your health by just meditating? It's a known method of relaxing the body and mind, but if done regularly, you'll find it actually benefits your overall health. You'll find that anxiety is less likely to affect you, and you won't immediately get anxious over small and unimportant things.

How you meditate depends on you, but many people enjoy listening to low music while they clear their mind and focus on their breathing. Emptying out your mind can be a clarifying experience, and it has the added benefit of calming you and making you feel more centered as you go about your day. If you suffer from anxiety and stress, meditation can help you reduce its effect on your body and calm you before you continue on with what you need to get done. It will also help you focus on the task at hand, instead of obsessing about what happened earlier.

If you find meditation confusing or difficult, consider using a guided meditation that you can listen to as you work on perfecting your technique. There are a number of free options on YouTube that can be used.

Meditation has the added benefit of using chanting or breathing techniques to help you relax, so you add another great method of activating your vagus nerve at the same time. You'll find that you have more energy and feel more balanced after a meditation session, too.

Prayer

Prayer isn't for anyone, but if you pray to someone or something, then this can help tone the vagus nerve, as well. The act of praying is very much like meditation, and it can work similarly to meditation intoning the vagus nerve. When you pray, you are completely focused on prayer. This clears your mind and brings calmness, but it is more than just that.

Having a belief in a more powerful being or force than yourself can give hope and a feeling of security. These are two things that contribute to the wellbeing of your nervous system.

Visualization

Your mind is a powerful part of your body, and it isn't used as much as it could be to improve overall health. If you've never heard of visualization and body awareness, now is a great time to start practicing both. This can be done in conjunction with deep breathing and meditation if you like.

Basically, you will close your eyes and visualize or imagine your vagus nerve. Start from the top of the body and imagine it reaching out to your throat. Visualize it, helping you inhale and exhale, smoothly and perfectly. Imagine the nerve reaching out to the various organs. You may not be able actually to control these organs, but you can visualize them working perfectly.

You can also focus on your heartbeat and consciously try to slow it if you like. Just being aware of the beating is often enough to activate the vagus nerve, though. Likewise, focus on the digestive system and visualize it working perfectly. This can actually result in better function of the GI tract.

Focusing on your body and how the vagus nerve works throughout it can be very beneficial. Do this regularly for 10 minutes a day, and you will see a surprising improvement in organ function. You may not be able to control your organs consciously, but you can certainly affect their function with your mind.

Practice Generosity

Being generous is something that can also help stimulate your vagus nerve. Not only does this give you a nice dose of daily interaction with other people and boost your social quotient, but it's also a great way to feel good about yourself.

Generosity can look like anything that involves giving from yourself. You could give a panhandler some change, but it's not necessarily about offering money. Other ways to be generous include:

Giving your time: Help someone out with a chore, sit and talk with a lonely person, or just spend some time with someone. You could volunteer at a retirement home or just chat with a lonely person in the park. Offer your services at a soup kitchen or food bank, and you could make a big difference. There are plenty of opportunities to share your time.

Share your food: Do you have some extra snacks? Why not share with someone who needs a boost? You could easily make their day. It's worth bringing a little extra food with you when you are out and about or going to work so you can share. It's amazing how much better the day gets when you give someone a chocolate bar or packet of crackers.

Give a compliment: Even your words can be generous. Try giving out at least five compliments a day. You'll feel great, and the people receiving them will feel good, too. Look for opportunities to tell people something nice about themselves. Don't just focus on appearances, either, and you can compliment their inner beauty, too, and really make them feel great. In some cases, complimenting someone who is always grumpy or in a bad mood can even turn their day around.

Pay for the person behind you: In the drive-through or at a grocery store, pick up the tab for someone else, and make their day while boosting your vagal tone. You never know what someone else is going through, and you could easily change the course of their day while you're going about your regular routine.

Foster a pet: If you love animals, why not make room in your home for a rescue? You can either adopt the pet or give it a temporary, loving home until it can find it forever home. Pets also have warming, relaxing effect on people and can give you a lot more than you give them. Who knows, you may even end up with a failed foster, where you keep the animal you were supposed to give back later.

Let someone cut in line: While driving or standing in line, let someone move ahead of you. It literally costs you nothing but a few seconds or a minute, but it is a generous move that will improve both your moods. Instead of fostering rage and frustration, smile, wave that person ahead, and increase that vagal tone.

There are few opportunities to be generous all around us. It doesn't have to be a grand gesture, but even little things can help change the course of someone's day, including yours. In addition, you'll get the added benefits for boosting your vagal tone.

Stretches

There's something to be said for stretching out your body and improving your health. Studies show that stretching can not only activate the vagus nerve but causes the release of GABA and acetylcholine, which work to reduce inflammation throughout the body. Since inflammation can be a bad thing if you have too much of it, it's important to keep that to a minimum. You can do that naturally just with some easy stretches.

There are a number of stretches you can do on your own, but those that engage the areas your vagus nerve reaches are most helpful. Any torso stretches or movements that engage the pelvis or neck can be good for getting the vagus nerve involved. You can also find videos on YouTube with stretches specifically designed to improve vagal tone.

While regular stretches can be useful, many people find it helpful to take up yoga. Yoga combines stretching with breathing, both of which activate the vagus nerve. You can take any type of yoga, but those that use Ujjayi breathing are particularly effective. In addition to breathing and stretching, yoga is often seen as a form of meditation, so the activity is even more beneficial for building that connection in the body and mind.

Joining a class can also help you by providing some real-life accountability. You won't want to skip the class if you paid for it, and even if it's free, you will find that working with others to improve your body is a great way to get in those social bonds and make new friends. For some people, it's also just easier to work out with someone else. You will find that stretching is quite the workout on its own, so get ready to really put those muscles to work.

Create a Routine

You need to be activating your vagus nerve on a daily basis, and the best way to do that is to simply incorporate the methods in these chapters into your daily routine. Make a schedule that includes as many methods of activating the nervous system as possible.

First, look at your schedule as it is today. You probably already have a routine, since most people are creatures of habit. So, when you wake up in the morning, you might shower, dress, then have breakfast, brush your teeth, and commute to work. Whatever your routine is, you can adjust it to include more opportunities to stimulate vagal tone and boost it.

In our example routine, you can easily change it up and add to the existing activities. For example:

Shower - instead of taking a regular shower, turn your water to cold and do a little cold exposure. You can also sing or hum while in the shower, to activate the vagus nerve via your throat and vocal cords.

Get dressed - do some jumping jacks or stretches before you pull on your clothes, and you'll get extra benefits. It doesn't have to be a long workout, just a few stretches to get things activated.

Eat breakfast - Take the time to really appreciate your food and feel gratitude for it. Chew slowly, experience the flavors and textures, and generally make breakfast about truly appreciating what you have. If you have loved ones, this is a good time to make eye contact and engage socially.

Brush teeth - gargle the rinse water after you brush your teeth, and you'll immediately activate the vagus nerve.

Commute to work - Sing, chant, or hum as you drive in the car. This is a good time to be generous, as well. You can easily let someone merge in front of you and take the time to smile at others as you drive. It doesn't have to be a huge gesture, but even the little things make a difference.

As you can see, it's fairly easy to incorporate these activities into your daily routine. It's just a little bit of adjustment, and you immediately turn each activity into something beneficial. Not only are you cleaning your teeth, but you're also toning your vagus nerve. When you associate specific actions with your daily routine, it becomes easier to remember them and to continue using these techniques each day.

You can also make a point of hugging each family member before you leave the house and when you come home, greeting your co-workers with a smile, and being generous to others as you go about your day. Lunch or breaks make a good time for a short meditation session, and you can eat with others to increase your social interactions.

Once you've mapped out your day, you'll see that there are plenty of opportunities to boost your vagal tone throughout the day. Doing so consciously will help you start adding more and more specific actions into your routine.

Timing: How Much Stimulation is Needed?

You've been reading throughout this book about how to stimulate your vagus nerve and how important it is to tone it, but how much time is really needed? Unfortunately, there is no one answer to this question. There are so many factors involved that it really depends on the person.

Every single person is different, and the amount of damage and the level of vagal tone will vary from person to person. What you need is completely different from what I need. For myself, I needed to do quite a bit. I'd spent years in pain, with the poor vagal tone, and it had only gotten worse over the years, plus I had nerve damage to contend with. But that's not the case for everyone.

If you're not sure how much to start with, aim for 20 minutes in the morning and evening. You can incorporate more activities into your daily routine, of course, but there should be roughly 10-20 minutes morning and night of specific vagal toning activities.

Studies with the vagus nerve stimulator showed that it didn't improve vagal tone when the nerve was stimulated constantly. It turned out to be more effective, stimulating it just several times a day. Keep this in mind as you go about your daily routine and make sure that you do something to activate your nerve every couple of hours.

It's very important that you set up a routine because without it, you'll likely forget to do anything, and that can only cause you to continue suffering. They say it takes 21 days to create a habit, and once you have established a habit, you can continue to do it without even thinking about it.

Decide what you want your habit to be and get

started today. The longer you wait, the more you have to deal with ongoing pain and symptoms that could be lessened if you just took action. While it does require time to build vagal tone and repair nerve damage, if you start today, you can look forward to experiencing relief sooner.

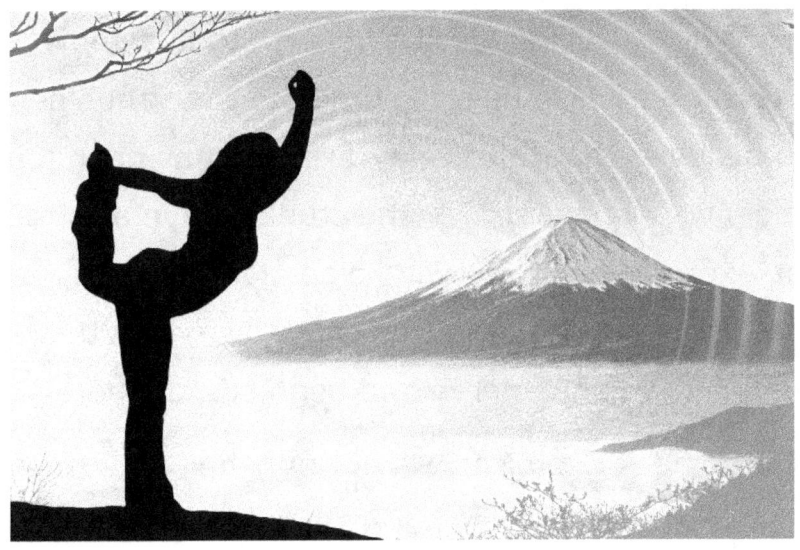

CHAPTER 20
VAGUS NEVER HEALING WITH NATURAL BODY EXERCISES.

Exercise is a very important part of living a healthy lifestyle. However, studies show that it may also help to stimulate the vagus nerve. It is believed that this is why exercise has been found to help with relaxation. Some studies have also found that exercise can help with digestion issues as well. What they found during that study was that this was because the vagus nerve had been stimulated.

These neck exercises will not only help to stimulate and activate your vagus nerve, but they are also going to help relieve the muscle tension in your back and neck. This is very helpful if you spend your day sitting at a desk looking at a computer.

Did you know that all exercise is going to help you to stimulate the vagus nerve? While it is very important for you to practice yoga and meditation in order to get the most benefits. All mild exercise is going to help to activate the vagus nerve.

How to Start Exercising

We all know how important exercise is to our health, but it may be even more important now that we understand how it affects the vagus nerve. Once you begin exercising, you are going to start to see so many benefits that you never thought were possible. However, finding the time to exercise each day is going to take some work, and making sure that you stick to your exercise routine is going to take some discipline.

If you have thought about beginning to exercise in the past but haven't been able to figure out how to start, don't worry, you are not alone.

The first thing that you need to think about when you decide that you want to start exercising is why? Do you want to exercise to lose weight? To feel better? To stimulate the vagus nerve and improve your health?

It is important that you know why you want to exercise because there are going to be times when you are going to want to give up. Reminding yourself why you started in the first place is a great way to keep yourself motivated.

The next thing that you want to think about is what type of exercise you want to do. If you are exercising in order to stimulate the vagus nerve, you do not have to take part in extremely intense workouts. Instead, simply going for a walk once a day, taking part in aerobic exercises, strength training, or focusing on balance or flexibility are all going to benefit you.

You can do these individually, or you can do a combination of any of them. For example, a person may choose to practice yoga and aerobic exercise. You can do whatever you want, just make sure that it is something that you are going to enjoy.

Now that you know why and what, you need to make sure that you are healthy enough to do the activities that you have chosen. Make sure that you talk to your doctor and tell them what you are planning. If, for example, you are not healthy enough right now to start aerobic exercise, your doctor is going to be able to suggest something more suitable. Don't give up though, as your body adjusts to the exercise and your vagus nerve is stimulated, you will be able to do those things that you want. You just have to work up to it.

This is also going to ensure that you are not creating any illusions in your head about the results that you are going to see. Your doctor is going to be able to explain to you how much exercise you should start with and how often you should do it.

Next, it is time for you to create a plan. You should make sure that the steps are going to be easy for you to follow and that they are going to help you improve your fitness level. Let's be honest, and if we are going to exercise in order to stimulate the vagus nerve, we might as well get the most out of it, right?

What is your goal? Do you want to run a 5k? Do you just want to be able to run? Do you want to lose weight so that you can get off of the oxygen? These are all great goals, and they are going to help keep you motivated as you work toward them. When you take a look at these goals, they may seem unattainable, and they are right now. You are not going to run a 5k if you can't run to the mailbox. However, you can break these goals down into much smaller goals, for example, running to the mailbox and back. Once you reach these small goals, you will be closer to reaching that big one.

Make exercise a habit. It is very important for you to stick to the routine of exercising. This is because you are only going to continue to see the benefits if you continue the action. While you are going to activate your vagus nerve by exercising, it is not a one-time thing. If it were, I would have given you a simple action that you could do once 44 pages ago, and that would have been the end of this book. Instead, it is something that we have to keep doing, stimulating the vagus nerve continually.

You can make exercising a habit by replacing one of your unhealthy habits with it. For example, if you normally watch television for an hour, replace 30 minutes of that with some exercise, or exercise while you watch television. Do whatever it takes to make this a habit. Many people find that they are better able to add exercise into their lives if they add it to something that they already do, such as watching television. You could easily watch television while exercising on a stationary bike. Personally, I like to listen to my podcasts or guided meditations while I exercise. I kill two birds with one stone, so to speak.

How much exercise should you try to do? You do not have to work out for hours each day. The truth is you probably are not going to be able to work out for an hour if you are just starting out. Instead, aim for a 30-minute workout five times per week.

If you can't do that, don't worry. Start as slowly as you need to start. If you are out of shape and the only thing you can do is five minutes of exercise twice a day. Do that! Work up to 10 minutes of exercise and then 20 and so on. As long as you are making progress and putting your best effort in, that is all that matters.

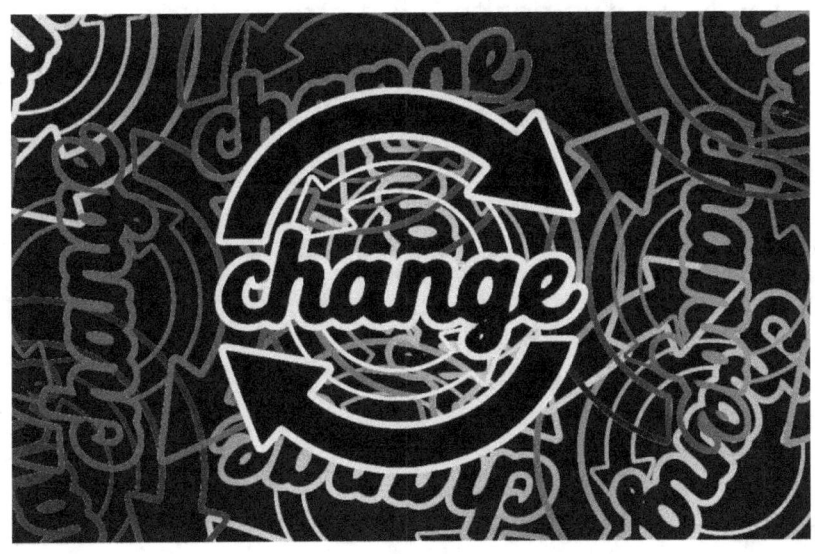

CHAPTER 21
PRACTICAL EXERCISES TO STIMULATE THE VAGUS NERVE

As we have read through the chapters, the vagus nerve is a sensitive nerve in our body. There are conditions and diseases prone to it when it is dysfunctional. Further, it is a powerful organ in the body to enhance that your body functions in the right way, that is healthy and strong. Further to this, you should not lose hope because there is a solution to your problem. The solution to the vagus nerve is stimulation. This chapter goes further to inform you of ways that your vagus nerve can be stimulated to enhance it to its maximum functional potential.

Neuro-Facial Release

This is otherwise known as myofascial release. If you have experienced pains and injuries, there is a likelihood that you have come across this therapy. This can be analyzed as a developed version that people opt to take in place of massage therapy and the common physiotherapy.

So, What Is Myofascial Release?

This is a practical guided methodology that assesses the entire body to heal the reason for the manifestations, regardless of whether it be in, snugness, and so forth. Myofascial Release endeavors to accomplish torment free, effective development designs, through arrangement and adjusting of the body. This type of treatment controls the body's sash, a dainty connective tissue that keeps running from the highest point of the head to the tip of the toes on a continuous web. It encompasses every one of the parts, lymph and veins, the nerves, the mind and spinal rope, and each muscle in the body. All development includes muscle and sash the which is the fascial framework.

Fascial limitations are regions of strain and snugness in the body's sash. Normally the fascia is entirely adaptable; however, this can turn out to be tight and inflexible with damage or stress – never again appropriately moving. These limitations and snugness in fascial and connective tissues can confine the body's development, adaptability, and capacity. They may cause strong brevity and snugness, which can cause torment by putting pressure on muscles or potentially joints. Confinements in the sash may likewise make limitations bloodstream, organ capacity, and nerves.

Any snugness and limitation in the fascia can realign the body. Consider a weaved cover or sweater – when one join gets stretched, the remainder of the encompassing lines likewise get stretched and twisted and are never again adjusted. This 'pulling' can make an individual abuse a hip since they are endeavoring to make up for the snugness and limitation in their development. For instance, fascial confinement of the internal thigh can haul the pelvis twisted, changing the situation of the spine and head, making a headache. Direct treatment of the migraine will just yield transitory outcomes; the first region of damage and the arrangement of the pelvis must be tended to when there is the release of fascial restriction their various things that happen in your body. First, there is the restoration of movement, the body is aligned properly, the body becomes much more flexible, there is increased circulation of blood and functioning of the organs, there is a change of postures and movements, and also the inflammation in the body reduces. Just before we look at a practical guide on performing neuro facial release, let me inform you how the restrictions come about.

In your day to day activities, you experience anxiousness and things that give you restriction in the body! Regardless of the amount we stretch and exercise, we as a whole have different development designs that bring about limitations. Notwithstanding, just when these confinements begin to meddle with our regular day to day existence (for example, cause torment or trouble moving), we start looking for medication.

Confinements can likewise shape because of injury, dull pressure damage, scarring, fiery responses, the impacts of gravity on an ineffectively adjusted body, and the stressors of daily life would all be able to make limitations inside the fascial framework. These confinements cause torment and firmness, making it hard for one to move and denying somebody from accomplishing those things they are interested in doing.

Step-by-Step Guide to Doing Myofascial Release

As we have seen above, therapy is an important exercise in stimulating your nerves. You should note that it is mostly done by specialists such as massage therapists or physiotherapists.

- The specialist starts by putting some pressure on your body
- They then engage stress and motion to stimulate and release fascial tensions and the restrictions that your body has formed.
- Depending on the needs of the body, the fascial release pressure varies. It can be heavy or light.

Further, you are advised to try these exercises;

- Ensure that you engage in exercises that stretch you for not less than 10 minutes
- Try manual therapy that induces your movement
- You should try to roll out the restricted

spots for example foam rolling

- Ensure that you make time to visit the sauna. There has been researching that has proved health benefits.
- Do some yoga
- Keep yourself hydrated
- You are advised to consult a professional if you do not know what to do by yourself

You may wonder, when is the right time for you to perform this therapy. Here is the detail:

Myofascial discharge can be successful in treating torment, which has recently been inert to different medications. Myofascial discharge specialists evaluate the entire body, instead of simply the region of agony. At the point when the patients have a feeling that they need an increasingly thorough take a gander at treatment, they frequently seek after myofascial discharge. Myofascial discharge can likewise enable the body to work all the more productively in increasingly thorough types of activity as it can give better versatility, quality, adaptability, and development.

Individuals who are encountering ceaseless and relentless agony additionally and frequently experience results, particularly those with fibromyalgia. This is because Myofascial discharge is extremely successful in treating irritation. Much of the time, an individual's sensory system can end up easily affected after damage or injury to the body. This outcome in an intensification of an individual's torment from muscle pressure and fascial confinements/. Myofascial discharge can quiet down the aggravation this torment enhancement causes to the sensory system. By attempting to assuage these confinements through these delicate systems, the body can discharge this strain and diminishing an individual's general torment.

Numerous individuals with injury likewise see myofascial discharge as an exceptionally viable treatment intending to their manifestations. Master-level myofascial specialists also have to prepare in helping the psyche and body in sensorimotor handling. Sensorimotor handling endeavors to change perception in the cerebrum by tending to the indications in the body. By diminishing aggravation and strain in the body through myofascial discharge, the mind can process psychological stressors all the more successfully all things considered in a more settled, less on edge state. For instance, following a day of unwinding, would it say it is a lot simpler to feel in a great and superior place in yours?

Massage for Migraines

A massage is a word that incorporates an assortment of strategies utilizing contact to press, rub, or control the skin, muscles, ligaments, and tendons. Back rub is utilized for a few wellbeing conditions and gives numerous medical advantages, including lessening pressure, torment, and muscle strain. Notwithstanding the medical advantages, numerous individuals discover back rub produces sentiments of the mind, solace, and association. There is some proof that back rub for headache sufferers may help diminish the number of migraines that attack them.

A study was done to test the effect and impact of massage for migraines among several individuals. The results of the study that had to undergo an observation revealed that; of the people who had the migraine massage, there was a drop in the pain and also revealed that they had a good sleep as compared to those who had not had the massage. Therefore, we can confidently conclude that migraine massage goes a long way in assisting you to improve your health and stimulates your nerves.

You need to know that you can perform self-massage for a migraine. There are specific points that have been proven to reduce pain and the symptoms that come along with the migraine such as nausea.

What Causes Headaches?

Scientists haven't recognized a complete reason for headaches. In any case, they have discovered some contributing elements that can trigger the condition. This incorporates changes in mind synthetic concoctions, for example, a lessening in levels of the serotonin, which is a chemical for the brain. Different elements that may trigger a headache include splendid lights, serious warmth, or different limits on climate, lack of hydration, changes in barometric weight, irregular hormones in ladies, for example, estrogen and progesterone vacillations during a monthly cycle, pregnancy, or menopause, overabundance stress, noisy sounds, serious physical movement, irregular eating habits, changes in rest designs, utilization of specific drugs, for example, oral contraceptives or nitroglycerin, uncommon scents, certain nourishments, smoking, liquor use, and voyaging.

If you experience a headache, your primary care physician may request that you keep a cerebral pain diary. Recording what you were doing, what nourishments you ate, and what prescriptions you were taking before your headache started can help recognize your triggers. Discover what else may cause or set off your headaches.

Nourishments That Trigger Headaches

There are foods or nourishment fixings that might be bound to trigger headaches than others. These may include liquor or stimulated beverages, nourishment added substances, for example, nitrates (an additive in relieved meats), aspartame (a fake sugar), or monosodium glutamate (MSG), tyramine, which normally happens in certain nourishments. Tyramine additionally is increased when nourishments are aged or kept for long. This incorporates nourishments like some matured cheeses, sauerkraut, and soy sauce. Be that as it may, continuous research is looking all the more carefully at the job of tyramine in headaches. It might be a cerebral pain defender in certain individuals instead of a trigger.

Step-by-Step Guide for Migraine Massage

- At the comfort of your house, dilute some peppermint oil and mix with the coconut oil.
- While it is fully mixed, use the tip of your first three fingers to touch on some oil (Do not smear all over your hand).
- Now massage the oil into the temples and your forehead
- Do it for about a minute.
- Make sure that you are relaxed, and your mind is not wandering.

Some patients may find it painful. In the case of this, you can add some peppermint and ensure that you are doing some breathing exercises. Make it a routine, and for sure, you will be fine.

Abdominal Massage

Abdominal massage is necessary for relieving pains and also stimulating your vagus nerve. The following exercise will assist you in having a great abdominal massage.

Step-by Step-Instructions to Conduct Abdominal Massage

This stomach rub system is anything but difficult to do at home in only a couple of minutes. It is ideal to complete this training on a vacant stomach, a couple of hours in the wake of eating. Start gradually and perceive how your body reacts.

Rests on a Relaxing Floor Tangle or a Bed

1. Spot your hand underneath your sternum or breastbone. Make delicate descending stroking developments moving your hand down toward your stomach area. Rehash this development for a couple of minutes, cycling one hand over the other in a regressive bicycle accelerating like movement.

2. Then, utilize your fingertips to make little roundabout movements on your belly. Start kneading the sides of your guts and gradually work your direction internal and descending. Go dynamically more profound, utilizing a firm yet the agreeable measure of weight. Proceed with this stomach rub for a few

minutes.

3. Finish the training with a couple of minutes of a delicate leaned back two-knee spinal contort present. This remedial yoga stance improves assimilation and energizes an opening inside the belt and stomach to enable you to develop your breath and actuate a mitigating unwinding reaction.

4. Lying on your back, breathe out as you press your lower back daintily into the floor or bed. Inhale here for a couple of minutes as your lower back opens. When you are prepared, delicately contract your muscular strength as you breathe in and twist your knees toward your chest.

5. Breathe out and bring your arms out to your side with your palms toward the floor, even with your shoulders.

6. On a moderate breath in, lift your heels somewhat higher than your knees, and afterward, as you breathe out gradually, lower the two legs to one side toward the floor.

7. Keep your knees at the degree of your hips, and your feet and knees stacked together. Rest in this position for 30 to 60 seconds

8. Keep taking moderate, full breaths as you delicately turn from one side to the other, following your breath.

Massage for Vagus Nerve Stimulation

The vagus nerve shouldn't be stunned into shape. It can likewise be conditioned and fortified like a muscle. Here are some straightforward things you can undertake that may improve your wellbeing, particularly:

1. **Energizing social circle** – An investigation had members ponder others while quietly rehashing positive expressions about loved ones. Contrasted with the controls, the members meditating demonstrated a general increment in positive feelings like quietness, delight, and expectation after finishing the class. These positive considerations of others prompted an improvement in the vagal capacity, as found in pulse changeability. The outcomes likewise demonstrated a more

conditioned vagus nerve than when just thinking.

2. **Cold** – Exposing yourself to something cold, for example, cool showers or face dunking, invigorates the nerve also. The previous research demonstrates that when your body changes with chills, your battle or flight (thoughtful) framework decays, and your rest and summary framework go up, and this is intervened by the vagus nerve. Any sort of intense cold introduction, including drinking super cold water, will expand vagus nerve actuation.

3. **Water gargling** – Another home solution for an under-animated vagus nerve is to gargle with water in your mouth. The gargle invigorates the pallet muscles, which are terminated by the vagus nerve. Commonly patients will tear up a piece, which is a decent sign, and if they don't, we prescribe that they do it normally consistently until they see that they do fire destroying a piece. This has been appeared to improve working memory execution promptly.

4. **Singing** – the singing of hymns, humming and also chanting, and peppy vigorous singing all expansion pulse inconstancy (HRV) in marginally various ways. Singing resembles starting a vagal siphon conveying loosening up waves, and singing as loud as possible works the muscles in the back of the throat to initiate the vagus. Singing as one, which is frequently done in houses of worship and synagogues, also builds HRV and vagus work. Singing has been found to build oxytocin, otherwise called the affection hormone, since it makes individuals feel more like each other.

5. **Back massage** – You can animate your vagus nerve by rubbing your feet and your neck along the carotid sinus, situated along the carotid supply routes on either side of your neck. A neck back rub can help decrease seizures. A foot back rub help can bring down your pulse and circulatory strain. A weight back rub can likewise actuate the vagus nerve. These back rubs are utilized to enable newborn children to put on weight by

animating gut work, to a great extent, interceded by initiating the vagus nerve.

6. **Chuckling** – Happiness and giggling are normal resistant sponsors. Chuckling likewise animates the vagus nerve. Research indicates how chuckling expands HRV in a gathering domain. There are different case studies of individuals blacking out from laughing too much, and this might be from the vagus nerve framework being animated excessively. Blacking out can come after chuckling, just as pee, hacking, gulping, or solid discharge, which are all aided along by vagus initiation.

7. **Yoga exercises** — This increases vagus nerve action and your parasympathetic framework when all is said in done. Studies have demonstrated that yoga builds a quieting synapse in your mind. Analysts trust it does this by "invigorating vagal afferents fibers which increase activity in the parasympathetic sensory system. This is particularly useful for the individuals who battle with uneasiness or despondency. Studies demonstrate that yoga additionally

can 'upgrade vagal tweak.'

8. Breathing Deeply and Slowly-Some neurons are found around your neck and heart are known as baroreceptors, which recognize circulatory strain and transmit the neuronal sign to your mind. This initiates your vagus nerve that associates with your heart to lower circulatory strain and pulse. Slow breathing, with a generic equivalent measure of time taking in and out, expands the affectability of baroreceptors and vagal initiation. Breathing around 5-6 breaths for each moment in the normal grown-up can be exceptionally useful.

9. **Exercise** – Exercises expand your mind's development hormone, bolsters your cerebrum's mitochondria, and helps turn around the psychological decrease. But at the same time, it's been appeared to animate the vagus nerve, which prompts valuable cerebrum and emotional well-being impacts. Mellow exercise likewise invigorates gut stream, which is the vagus nerve intercedes.

10. **Espresso Enemas** — Enemas resemble runs for your vagus nerve. Growing the gut

expands vagus nerve enactment, as is finished with purifications. This purging is cultivated by expanding the liver's ability to detoxify poisons in the blood and restricting them to the bile. All the while, the liver washes down itself as it discharges the dangerous bile into the little, at that point enormous, the digestive system for departure. The whole blood supply flows through the liver at regular intervals. By holding the espresso 12 to 15 minutes, the blood will circle four to multiple times for purging, much like a dialysis treatment. The water substance of the espresso invigorates intestinal peristalsis and purges the internal organ with the gathered harmful bile.

11. **Nirvana-**This wearable item sends a delicate electrical wave through the left ear channel to animate the body's vagus nerve while synchronizing with music, which thusly invigorates the arrival of synapses in the cerebrum that create a quieting sensation all through the body.

12. **Unwind** – Learning how to relax might be

the major thing to help keep your vagus nerve conditioned. This is because you free up your mind and let loose hence causing relaxation to the nerves too. Research shows that most loosening up exercises causes the vagus nerve to stimulate

Meditation

Meditation helps you to focus and become aware of your mind by focusing and helps in training attention, to have a result of a stable mind, and to have a clear mind. The primary thing to explain:

What we're doing here is going for care, not some procedure that mysteriously wipes your mind clear of the incalculable and unlimited contemplations that eject and ping always in our cerebrums. We're simply working on pointing out our breath, and after that, back to the breath when we see our consideration has meandered.

Get settled and get ready to be settled and relaxed for a couple of minutes. After you quit understanding this, you're going to just concentrate without anyone else common breathing in and breathing out of breath.

Concentrate on your breath. Where do you feel your breath most? Is it in your stomach? Or in your nose? Attempt to keep your consideration on your breath in and breath out.

What was the deal? To what extent would it say it was before your thoughts lost focus away from your breath? Did you see how bustling your brain was, even without you intentionally guiding it to consider anything specifically? Did you see yourself becoming involved with contemplations before you returned to understanding this? We regularly have little stories running in our mind that we didn't put there, similar to: "For example, you can be thinking, "why does the manager need to meet with me tomorrow?" "I could have gone shopping yesterday when there was an offer." "I must take care of certain tabs" or (the work of art) "I don't have the opportunity to sit still, because there is a lot that I need to attend to."

If maybe you encountered these sorts of interruptions as it happens to all of us most of the time, you've made a significant revelation: basically, that is something contrary to care. It's the point at which we live in our minds, on the programmed pilot, releasing our contemplations to a great extent, investigating, state, the future, or the past, and basically, not being available at the time. In any case, that is the place the vast majority of us live more often than not and pretty awkwardly, in case we're straightforward, correct? Be that as it may, it doesn't need to be like that.

We always train on care and attentiveness so we can figure out how to perceive when our psyches are doing their typical regular aerobatic exhibition, and perhaps take a delay from that for only a short time so we can pick what we'd like to concentrate on. Contemplation encourages us to have a lot more advantageous association with ourselves.

When we contemplate, we infuse extensive and enduring advantages to our lives. Furthermore, reward: you needn't bother with any additional rigging or costly participation.

Here are five motivations to ponder:

- Helps you recognize the pain that you are undergoing
- Helps in bringing down your pressure
- Helps you to have a great connection with yourself

- Helps you regain your focus

Step-by-Step Instructions to Meditate

The act of meditation is more straightforward and harder than a great many people think. Make sure that you are in someplace where you can unwind into this procedure, set a clock, and give it a shot:

- Sit down. Discover a spot to sit that feels quiet and calm to you.

- Set a period limit. In case you're simply starting, it can pick a brief timeframe, for example, five or 10 minutes.

- Have an awareness of your body. You can sit in a seat with your feet on the floor; you can sit freely leg over leg, you can bow, all are fine. Simply ensure you are steady, and in a position, you can remain in for some time.

- Feel your breath. Pursue the impression of your breath as it goes in and as it goes out.

- Notice when your mind has moved away from your focus. Your attention will probably leave different spots with the wind and the meander. Just restore your air attention when you're about to see your mind has meandered in no particular order, a moment, five minutes.

- Be kind to your meandering character. Try not to judge yourself or to determine the nature of the circumstances in which you end up lost. Simply return.

- That is, it! That is training. You leave, you return, and you attempt to do it as merciful as could be expected under the circumstances.

- Close with graciousness. When you're prepared, tenderly lift your look (if your eyes are shut, open them). Notice any sounds in nature. Notice how your body feels at this moment. Notice your musings and feelings.

Salamander Exercises

This exercise is meant to activate your joints and muscles hence stimulating your vagus nerve. This exercise is all-round helpful to your body because it connects your core, hip, and shoulder stability. You need to be ready for whole body activation. Let us get right in and learn the guide to doing these exercises.

Step one: Lay down, with your face facing down. Hold and lift yourself with your palms, forearms, and the left knee. Keep your toes pointed to the ground. Breathe in and the right leg up and stretch it to be straight

Step two: Breathe out as you get down slowly on your right side of the hip. While in this position

- Get control and get down
- Get to the ground with the outer part of your hip before your ankle and knee get down
- You will be able to go down to the ground with your foot right behind, as you progress and advance.
- As you go down, try to view your left shoulder.

Step three: Breathe in and lift your right leg again, just as in the first step

- Let your toes point to the ground
- Stretch your leg with your right glute

Step four: Breathe out and return to the ground with a lift on your arms and palms. Repeat the exercise with your left side. Doing this exercise will help stimulate your nerves and also bring back your mindfulness.

Angle Pose

On the next exercise, we shall focus on the angle pose. As you are aware, all these exercises are guides into helping your vagus nerve. Eight-edge posture is significantly less terrifying to start tinkering around with than a portion of the other arm adjusts, as you start from a situated position as opposed to descending into it. Also, a great deal like in shoulder press present where your legs are crushing your shoulders, in eight-edge, you have your thighs pressing together over your arm to help hold you up, giving you an additional layer of help, so it's not only the arms and the abs.

Step by Step Guide

- **Step one:** Lay down on your back. Start by stimulating your hips and go into the baby rest position, with the knees on your elbow and legs up above your face. You can try to lift your legs one at a time.

- **Step two**: Get up slowly and stand up. Bend forward with your bums up. Go on to fold your hands as you touch opposite elbows. Start swaying from side to side.

- **Step three**: Stand up and spread your legs apart. Stretch your right hand to touch your left ankle and your left hand to grab the left ankle. As one touches the other, open up your free arm into the air up the ceiling.

- **Step four:** stand up. Then squat. From that position, stretch out your left leg to the side straight. Keep your hands on the ground. Do that to the opposite side as you move your hands. Repeat several times up to five times and rest on the part that you feel good.

- **Step five**: At this point, your body has been warmed up and stimulated. Have a sit on your mat and spread out your legs. Step by step lift and fold one leg towards your chest. Stay for five minutes and alternate.

- **Step six:** When flexible enough with your right leg up, bring it up to rest on your shoulder. This needs you to be very flexible. If it brings a little bit of trouble, do it slowly at your comfort. With time you will manage it.

- **Step seven:** Cross your legs and let your ankles crossed. Put your arm in the middle of your thighs and roll the shoulder while in between. This is a position that requires flexibility, ensure that you allow yourself to adapt slowly.

- **Step eight:** Hold on to the ground with your hands, still while one arm protrudes between your legs as you lift your bums. Transfer your weight to your hands.

Congratulations. You can always try this angle poses for your muscle stimulation. This pose further helps you to strengthen your knees, legs, and ankles while also having an impact in your body by stretching and toning up your muscles.

Reclined Angle Pose

The reclined angle pose is a favorite to many. It is easy after a long day and also as an entry point into your exercises. It helps bring you to attention and mindfulness. This posture makes an inactive, delicate stretch for the internal hips and crotch, which can be left dismissed in progressively overwhelming, streaming guides. Because of the therapeutic idea of the posture, it can likewise alleviate side effects of pressure, a sleeping disorder, mellow melancholy, monthly cycle, or menopause. Leaned back Bound Angle Pose is additionally a phenomenal posture for pregnancy, as it opens up and empowers the pelvic organ.

Step-by-Step Guide into This Exercise

- Start by lying down on your back while relaxed, stretch your legs, and relax your arms by the sides. Make sure that the palms of your hands are facing up.

- While at that position, fold your knees in such a position that will cause your feet soles to touch. Your little pinky toe should be on the mat. You've achieved that, good! Now let your legs fall open and just rest for the law of nature to support your leg's weight.

- Depending on your weight and flexibility, you may feel very tight around your hip or groin. If you feel this, you can extend your feet further from your body but if you are comfortable, bring the feet closer and cause an in-depth stretch

- Now, I need you just to relax the shoulders from the ears and cause your whole body to have an in-depth into the mat. Depending on your body and comfort, stay in that position from two to five minutes.

- To finish up with the pose, take the hand palms on the thighs facing the outer part and have a gentle folding of your legs. Now bring the soles of your feet to rest on the ground. Hold your knees to the chest and allow the relaxation of your low back.

You can always do this exercise when you need to. It is an easy way to relax after a long day and also bring focus into your body mind and soul.

Some Tips as You Undertake the Exercise

It is advised that you have your arms wide enough as you feel comfortable because the larger the room you give on the arms and body, the more you enlarge the shoulder bones and permit the back of the body to unwind. A superb method to help yourself in this posture is to put some pillow, blanket or bolsters under you. These items will contribute to helping you feel relaxed and be profoundly remedial.

The greater part of us tends to be tight in the hips and crotch from sitting at a work area throughout the day. As opposed to opposing the inconvenience, breathe in and send your breath and your understanding even into the most rigid pieces of yourself they need love as well! Relinquishing strain in one zone of the body can some of the time in a roundabout way send pressure somewhere else. As you stay in this posture, make sure to keep the jaw loose, the breath enduring, and to keep your mind and heart open to receive all the transformation.

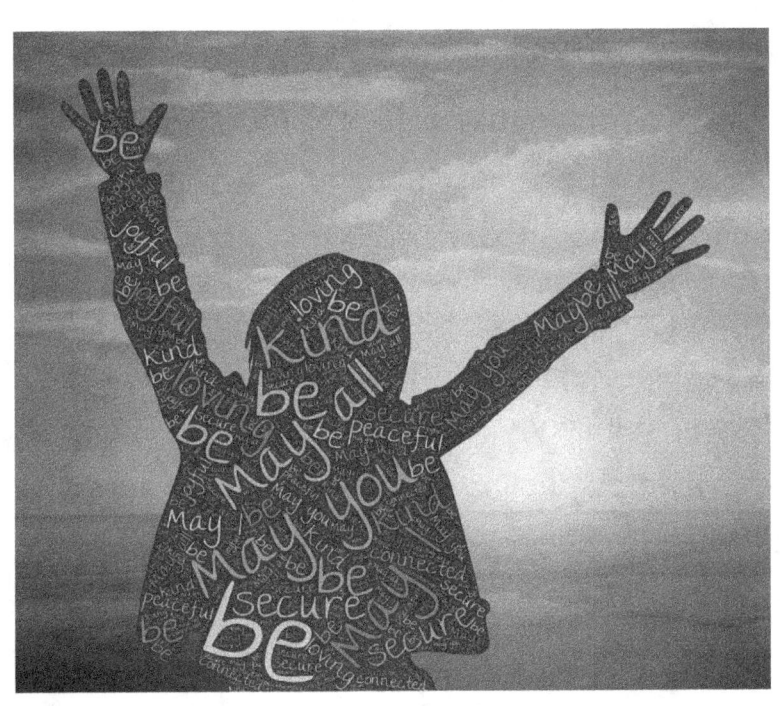

CHAPTER 22
WINDOW OF TOLERANCE

Your Optimal State

The vagal ladder is one way of describing where we are on the scale of safety. Another one that may resonate more with some of us is the window of tolerance.

Imagine a wave. The crest of the wave, the very top, is hyperarousal – that state where a person feels anxious, panicky, has a high startle reflex, and an uneasy antsy feeling in their stomach. We have all seen it, the teenagers watching a scary movie in the dark and someone walks in on them unexpectedly. They all jump and scream, maybe knock over a lamp in the process. This is because they have been placed in a state of hypervigilance by the movie they were watching. Staying in this state for too long can also lead to chronic pain, sleeplessness, and hostility.

The bottom of the wave, the low trough, is hypoarousal – that state where a person feels depressed, isolated, has a flat or blank affect, may feel tired all the time, and suffer from chronic fatigue. I am sure you have seen people in this state as well – perhaps after the loss of a loved one or has a major life disappointment.

In between these two extremes is a quiet middle ground, that area where we all want to live. When going through something difficult, it is normal for our bodies to activate its defensive systems. What we don't want is to live in those defensive states for too long. We want to come back to that window of tolerance in a relatively short time where we can function in a healthy way. We can know that we are still functioning in this optimal space when we are able to engage socially, willing to reach out to those around us, and ask for help.

Trauma kicks us out of this optimal state and into either the over-vigilant state or when that is left unaddressed, may lead to us falling lower into depression. This can be demonstrated in terms of a wave-like effect. We live life in that window of tolerance, but then a trauma happens, kicking us into the hyper-arousal, or activated state. The parasympathetic system, largely the vagus nerve, does its job and brings us down from that overly activated state, but if we do not address the initial trauma, then the vagus nerve can do too good of a job, our body becoming lethargic and falling into depression, what many people describe as feeling dead inside. Left unchecked, we may unconsciously try to counter this deadness inside with risky behaviors in order to try to kick us back up to a more activated state, leading to potentially dangerous situations.

A safer way of regulating ourselves is necessary, which is why we need to learn about the regulation of the vagus nerve.

Vagal Brake

Vagal brake is a term that refers to the moment when a person is able to stop the sympathetic nervous system from overriding their rational thought patterns. When the vagal brake is strong, the person is able to successfully handle stress and irritation without either going into hyper-vigilance or swinging down into a depressed state. When this vagal brake is weakened or non-existent, the person is unable to process stressors or at least is greatly hindered in handling them. This might be someone who flies off the handle at the least provocation, or they run from even minor confrontation. In severe cases, you may even see someone completely ignore a person who is trying to have a dialogue with them if there is even a hint of confrontation there.

We have all been on the brink... that moment when we see the conflict in our own heart. Maybe the first simmers of an angry retort or the grinding irritation of being cut off in traffic. We have had that moment when someone jumps out at us from around a corner trying to scare us, and the first instinct is to pull an arm back and punch the person. Our fight mode has been activated through the sympathetic nervous system.

When we bite our tongue and do not respond to the angry yell when we hold ourselves back from making a rude gesture at the driver that cut us off in traffic when we hold back the punch from actually connecting with the nose of our friend who just startled us – those are indications of our vagal brake.

This is an important part of our neurological development, and it can save our lives if we let it. I once heard the story of a young woman driving down a busy freeway in afternoon traffic – crowded, but still moving at a good clip. Her two children were buckled into their car seats in the back, a six-year-old girl and a four-year-old girl. The mom was driving along, anticipating getting home and getting the girls a snack before her husband was due back home, when all of a sudden, a blood-curdling scream erupted from the backseat. Her youngest daughter had just hit the panic button in a big way, abject terror evident in her voice. This scream is the sort that will cause every adult, parent, or not parent, to jump into immediate action. It signals imminent danger, complete need for rescue, no questions asked. Immediately the mom was thrown hard into a sympathetic response.

The problem was the woman was driving her car down a crowded freeway at sixty miles per hour. Stopping was out of the question, swerving to the side of the road was definitely out of the question. Though her initial response was to grip the wheel and immediately swerve to the side of the road, the young mother was able to stop the progress of her hands just in time to keep the wheel steady. Her heart was racing, and her hands were sweaty, her breath was coming in gasps. Still, she managed not to push the gas pedal down harder or slam her foot onto the brake. After the initial pulse of strong energy, she was able to signal left, pull to the next lane, and off onto the shoulder of the road to safety.

Still breathing hard, hands still sweaty, the young mother was able to turn and calmly ask her daughter what had just happened and, thankfully, was also able to respond when her daughter pointed to a harmless spider walking across her foot appropriately.

Anxiety

Fear is a necessary neurological response. Without it, we do not recognize the danger and take the appropriate reaction to either ward off that danger or escape.

Anxiety is about more than just fear, though. The problem comes when our body does not recognize when that danger has passed or is not what the body assumes it to be. Our body can become trapped in that fear response, creating a sense of constant anxiety, even paranoia. Certain things can spark anxiety, growing from their gut as their dorsal vagus nerve tells their brain that something is wrong, even though the person can see that nothing around them is dangerous. This creates a sense of confusion and only adds to the anxiety.

Oftentimes the person is suffering from a weakened vagal brake, having a brain that has become used to the anxiety reaction. Those nerves learn to react that way, and eventually become wired together, creating a constant sense of anxiety. Sometimes the anxiety comes from a traumatic event, and anything that reminds them of that event then triggers the anxiety.

This is when panic attacks happen. Your body is so used to the anxiety taking over that you dread its approach. Your mind is so caught up in that anxiety and fear of the anxiety itself, that now your body reacts in a panic response – your body is afraid of its own reaction and is trying to flee. This is why grounding techniques are particularly helpful with anxiety and panic attacks.

We see now what happens when someone becomes stuck in the "on" position, outside of the window of tolerance at the top of the wave we described above, in the hyperarousal state.

Anxiety is a practiced response, and so the only way to overcome it is to reteach the neural pathways to respond in a quieter fashion to triggering stimuli.

There are various methods you can do to help yourself break out of the anxiety cycle at the moment.

For instance, counting backward from ten to one. It really does help. I have seen it work countless times.

Another method of breaking yourself out of the anxiety at that moment is to ground yourself in your five senses. Focus again on where your feet are touching the ground. Pick out a leaf on a nearby tree or search the ground for one of those pennies that people always drop. Try to figure out exactly what you can smell nearby. Perhaps you can smell a nearby bakery. What are they cooking that day? Perhaps you can smell a wet dog or a bed of roses in the garden. Determine what you are hearing nearby. Do you hear the sound of children playing or traffic going by? Soon you will feel the anxiety slipping away. Let it go. You will be safe without it.

Another method is to try a simple breathing exercise like this one. Breathe in for a count of four, hold your breath to the count of four, then breathe out to a count of four. After this, wait to a count of four, then repeat until you feel yourself calming again.

Sometimes the anxiety is crippling, creating a barrier for a person to lead the life they would like to lead. One thing that has been very effective for many people in this situation is to name your anxiety. Give it an actual person's name. Perhaps a character from a movie which you found particularly annoying. Welcome the now-named anxiety as if it were a real person. Invite it to walk alongside you, but not to dictate what direction you will go. Then decide where you will go next. Physically walk to that location. Practice taking charge of your anxiety as if it were a real person, and you had to put them in their proper place – a place not in charge of your life.

All of these methods call for the person to live again in a state of safety. Anxiety believes itself to be unsafe. You can convince it otherwise.

It is important to help ourselves have a healthy vagal brake, but in all honesty, we need each other to co-regulate effectively. We balance each other, as we will find out next.

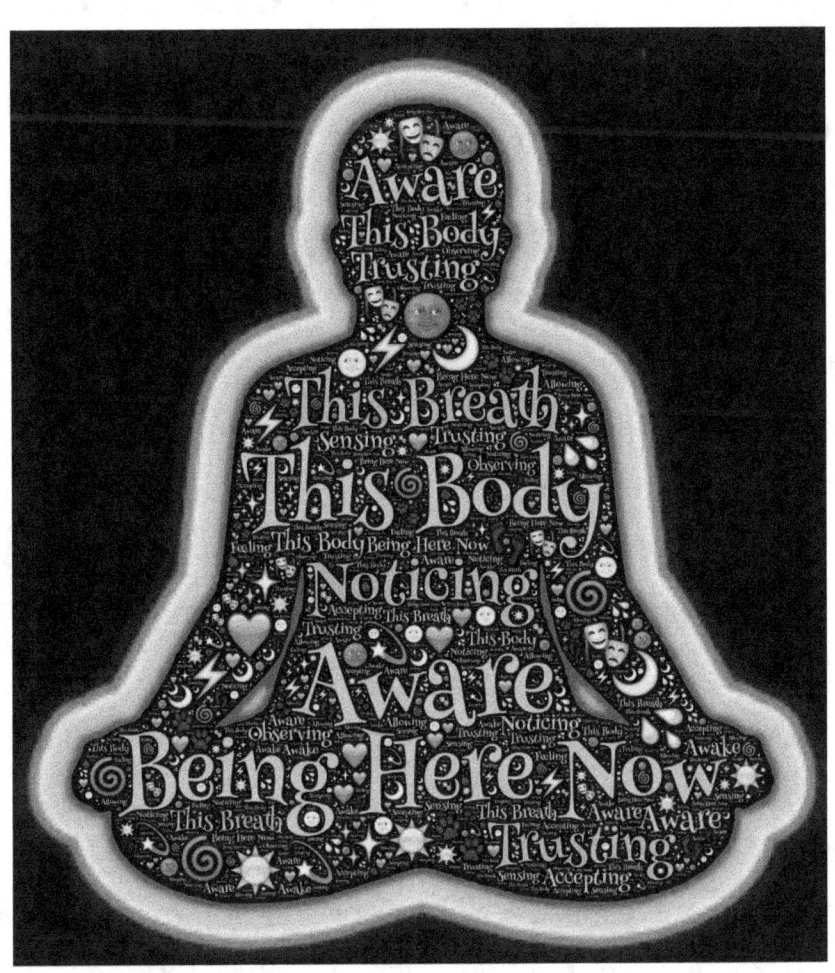

CHAPTER 23
BODY AND MIND CONNECTION

The profound idea that consciousness and matter are interwoven stems from an enlightened mind, as our individual consciousness is interwoven with our physical body. Our individual consciousness is the result of a coherent whole of the body (including the brain). Our individual consciousness is a byproduct of the quantum-interconnected whole of the body, which, in turn, is quantum-interconnected with the entire universe.

The tendons are comprised of twisted collections of collagen bundles, each of which is composed of collagen fibers. In other words, tendons are part of the connective tissue system or the liquid crystalline matrix. As connective tissue, our tendons are semiconductors and are able to conduct information, in addition to energy or electricity.

Another aspect of connective tissue (which includes muscles and tendons) is its piezoelectric properties. A piezoelectric substance can convert mechanical energy into electricity. The tendons' piezoelectric properties are nearly the same as those of a quartz crystal. By stretching the tendons in your body, you can thus convert mechanical energy into a DC field or direct current or chi, as it is referred to in TCM.

Many of the tendons in our body are components of the so-called meridians or energy channels. Stretching properly opens the meridians and allows the chi to flow freely. As for how opening the meridians can be understood, our insights are as follows:

As part of the connective tissue, meridians have a liquid crystalline structure. The higher the crystalline structure of the meridians, the better they convey energy and information.

Stretching all of the meridians can improve overall health. The main meridians are connected respectively to different organs of the body. Stretching a particular meridian improves the physical health of organs associated with that meridian. However, stretching all of the meridians makes the body more efficient, as doing so enhances the coordination of all of the organs. More open meridians increase intercommunication within the body and the efficiency of a whole coherent body.

Qigong practices include methods for leading or guiding the *Chi* with the mind. In principle, this practice is very simple. Whenever the mind or awareness focuses on the body, the chi follows. In other words, sensing a particular part of the body causes the chi to travel to that part of the body. Practically speaking; however, such practices should be conducted with the assistance of a master, as inexperienced individuals can disturb the natural flow of *Chi*.

The way of Tao is not a discipline, but rather refers to a spontaneity that emerges by going with the natural flow of things and the wholeness. The philosophy of Lao Tzu cannot be practiced. Whenever you attempt to practice it, you miss it. In fact, the philosophy of Tao is not actually a philosophy, but rather a natural way of living. We will continue to refer to it as a philosophy anyway. The philosophy of Tao differs from Taoism as a religion. The religious form of Taoism came into being approximately one hundred years after Buddhism was first imported to China.

However, the *Zhan Zuang* exercises cannot be

regarded as a true discipline, as they aim to open paths for chi to flow naturally by being in tune with the body as a whole. We do not aim to guide chi to a particular area of the body by stretching, but rather to create conditions that enable the natural flow of chi and that foster the body's wholeness. To add to others' hypotheses, we suggest that chi may serve as the direct current or DC field inherent in the liquid crystalline medium of connective tissues and the myelin sheath of nerves that enable instantaneous intercommunication throughout the body.

Not only do higher implicate orders organize the lower ones in physical reality, but the lower ones also influence higher orders. Thus, it doesn't matter whether or not you believe in Zhan Zhuang exercises; doing them will improve your consciousness.

CHAPTER 24
HOW PAIN, STRESS, AND ANXIETY AFFECT YOUR LIFE

How pain affects your life

At least 100 million Americans, or one in three, live with chronic pain. It's a debilitating condition that affects your ability to work, exercise, focus, relax, do basic household tasks, get a good night's sleep, and fully enjoy life.

Pain can affect your life in numerous ways. If you are a professional and have to go to work, if you experience pain, your work is affected. You will not be able to concentrate on finishing your tasks if something is wrong with you. If you are sick, you have to be absent for treatment or rest. Either way, your work is still affected. If you are a parent, how can you take care of your kids if you are hurt? Pain is, of course, a natural stimulus that should not be taken for granted. The more you ignore the pain, the worse your situation may become.

If pain is chronic, it has a detrimental effect on the everyday life of the person. It affects the patient's ability to perform natural functions and responsibilities. Physical activities are limited.

Chronic pain affects you physically and psychologically. It limits what you can do. It interferes with your ability to work, play with your children or grandchildren; it also diminishes your ability to take care of your own self. When these happen, pain causes you to feel useless and incompetent, making you succumb to a depressed state. People with chronic pain often experience irritability, anger, depression, and difficulty in concentrating. It becomes as debilitating as the pain itself.

It pressures the person while he is trying to hide the pain and forces himself to cover the handicap by a sense of forged well-being to be functional.

Chronic pain is unpredictable. It is sometimes mild, and other times, it is unbearable. When a person is in pain, his perception of things is obscured, and his responses are slow. This is the stage where a person's personality does not reflect on the outside.

Pain causes sleeplessness and mood swings. Chronic pain leads to painful depressions and helplessness, which, in turn, leads to suicidal tendencies, anxiety, and panic disorders.

If you're in chronic pain, do you notice the effects that it has on your mood and ability to live a normal life? If you have a loved one who suffers from chronic pain, have you noticed changes in them since their pain began?

Chronic pain has become a large-scale public health issue that dramatically worsens the quality of life for many people and creates a sizable and growing financial drain on our health care system. The core of the issue is that the medical community does not know how to address the underlying cause of most chronic musculoskeletal pain. Why are drugs and surgery, which are effective roughly 50% of the time, their go-to treatments? The answer that "these are the best solutions we have" is simply not good enough anymore.

People who are in painful situations are always misunderstood. Oftentimes, their real perception and intentions are not reflected on the outside. Their ways of coping with pain are essentially vital to how people view them. Their view of life is also affected. Those who suffer from serious illnesses perceive life as something they have to live to the fullest as their time is already counted and the likes. Some also become hopeless and afraid of the things to come.

To shift out of the surgery-focused trend, some big changes are necessary. Doctors must be educated about the effectiveness of preventive care compared to surgery, and communicate this to their patients. Insurance companies must start covering more types of preventive care. And as a patient, you need to do your part by educating yourself about your condition and getting opinions from multiple doctors. You should also recognize that in many cases, there are no magic pills or surgeries that will cure your pain forever. You must put in the work required to take care of yourself on a daily basis so that you can get out of and stay out of pain.

Imaging studies show that regions of the brain involved in making emotional decisions are also involved in chronic pain. To explore this connection, researchers at Northwestern University Medical School and SUNY Upstate Medical University paired chronic back pain patients with healthy control subjects on the Iowa Gambling Task, a card game that measures emotional decision-making abilities. The chronic pain patients performed poorly compared to the control subjects, showing the negative impact chronic pain has on your ability to make decisions.

Another major challenge is that people suffering from chronic pain tend to feel like they have no understanding or control over their pain. Despite all that modern medicine knows about the human body, the medical community still understands relatively little about pain—so much so that 85% of lower back pain sufferers receive no definitive diagnosis.

How Stress and Anxiety Affects Your Body and Life

There can be situations when you just cannot act like before you used to because now anxiety has taken a grip on you. It is the feeling of being afraid of the unknown. In a broader sense, anxiety comes in different forms, sometimes feeling worried, apprehensive, being nervous, or plainly everything going out of control. Severe forms of anxiety can be extremely devastating and can have a great impact on your life and health.

Fear and panic are natural human emotions. Everyone has felt anxious for one reason or another.

It is the feeling of worry, apprehension, or panic in response to certain situations, which is usually unsafe or uncomfortable.

Anxiety is a basic human emotion. Generally speaking, it is healthy and manageable to a certain degree. Because everyone experiences anxiety, it can be challenging to recognize and accept anxiety as a problem. However, if you just ignore the symptoms of anxiety, you miss the chance to understand your life and yourself better. If you try to understand what your anxiety is telling you, you will have a better chance of overcoming the problem. In effect, you get to enjoy a better quality of life.

Is your anxiety helping you, or has it become excessive and detrimental? We'll now try to learn more about anxiety and what you can do to help control the problem.

There are several 'listed' disorders that are all classified as 'anxiety.' Depending on the duration of the anxiety and its severity, it can actually lead to physical symptoms. When it manifests physically, it can cause the person to feel worn out, rundown, fatigued, it can cause pain in muscles and joints, it can lead to an increased risk of getting sick, and it can even increase the risk of heart attack, stroke, and a number of other health emergencies.

There are probably plenty of things that you have gone through in your life that caused you some level of worry. Maybe you had a test in high school that worried you. Even if you studied and felt confident that you knew the material, you might have worried about that test.

Maybe it kept you from getting a good night's sleep right before that test. Would that be considered anxiety?

It all depends. Since it interfered with your ability to sleep, some people could have been diagnosed as having mild anxiety. But most likely, once the test was over, you were able to get back to your normal routine and didn't worry about it anymore, and that wouldn't be classified as anxiety, more like stress.

We all experience stress throughout our life. It's quite natural and normal, but when you begin to worry excessively about certain things, especially things that you cannot control, then it becomes a problem.

As you deal with stress on a regular basis, whether it's because of financial pressures, schooling, relationship problems, worries about your job or finding work, or anything else, it can develop into anxiety over time.

What usually happens is that the worry starts to consume your thoughts. You begin thinking about the challenges you're facing on a regular basis. You could be thinking about the rent that's late while driving home from work, knowing you can't possibly pay it right now.

You could be worried about the company you work for downsizing. You might be concerned about your adult child's well-being because he's out partying every night, doesn't seem to be taking any responsibility for his life, is getting himself into debt, and nothing you say or do –aside from paying those bills for him-is making a difference.

When you try to fall asleep at night, when the TV is off, and everything is quiet, you can't shut the worry and stress off. You keep turning those fears over and over in your mind.

At some point in the middle of the night, you might finally drift off to sleep, but the alarm blares just two or three hours later. Now you're tired and have the deal with another day like that.

Multiply that night after night, and the anxiety will continue to build even more because now, you're trying to focus at work, impress the boss, or getting impatient with people around you.

You might snap at somebody then feel bad about it right away, and that's going to make things worse in your mind. Eventually, you may feel tightness in your chest, shortness of breath at times, and have a difficult time getting anything done.

Over time you might withdraw from some of the activities you used to enjoy because you're spending all of your time worrying about everything, even though you're not actually able to do anything about them.

In time, you're living a completely different life with little to enjoy. That can lead to depression and a general state of worry about many other things, even those things that weren't a major concern for you in the past.

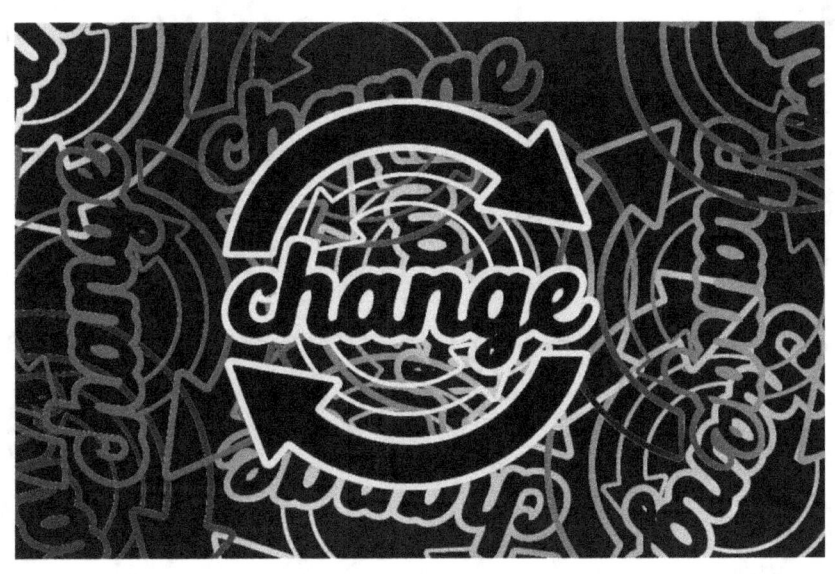

CONCLUSION

Sometimes, and maybe more often than we actually care to admit to ourselves, the easily accessible power that the vagus nerve holds in order to reduce inflammation and anxiety gets underestimated and overlooked as a method of balanced treatment for the body.

We are often far too quick to reach for Ibuprofen and Prozac and don't always realize that we have to tools to balance our lives right in the palm of…well, not our hands specifically, but in our nervous system and waiting to be used.

You could almost go as far as to say that the vagus nerve has its own type of 'yin yang' factor to it.

By this, I mean that with the vagus nerve, we have both the sympathetic and parasympathetic nervous systems that are polar opposites in what they do. On the sympathetic side, you have you fight or flight mode that gives you a burst of adrenaline and cortisol in order to pounce on whatever may be about to attack you (currently in my case, a spider that is eyeballing me from the wall opposite where I am sitting), while on the other hand, your parasympathetic nerve which allows you to relax and lower your breathing and heart rate after the burst of energy previously felt. (I think I will name him Michael). So when Michael decides to shimmey his way back out the window to his little spider family, my parasympathetic nervous system can kick in and allow me to breathe again!

The tug of war in a push and pull fight between these two sides of the nervous system thus creates the ultimate balance within your body with homeostasis.

If we go back in time, and I mean many, many years, we could look at the possibilities from an evolutionary perspective, too. We could probably say that our ancestors relied on the sympathetic nervous system in order to get their instincts for hunting as well as to stay safe against any enemies that could potentially attack them or steal their food supply.

On the other hand, the parasympathetic nervous system probably allowed others in the family tree to bond between and make sure that the family was cared for as well as to ensure the procreation of the next generation and build supportive communities amongst themselves.

Sadly, for the rest of us, the 21st century has caused a lot of change over a short period of time that we, as the next generation, have had to struggle to keep up with the times.

This, in turn, is causing our systems to completely short circuit more often than not, and we have to go all out to keep the balance necessary for our body's survival. Our nervous systems have no idea what is going on these days! Recent studies have shown that social media and other modern-day technological factors are causing far more social isolation, anxiety, depression, and feelings of being unworthy of love. On top of that, we have made it a habit to have "every man for himself" becoming the norm, which can also throw off some people's fight and flight responses, as you don't have anyone that you can turn to should you need physical or emotional help.

Fortunately, the last few generations have figured out how we can use the vagus nerve to our benefit, and this is slowly developing its way into a full rolling therapy treatment for many people. Researchers are still to this day and minute finding new ways to use the vagus nerve to our advantage and tweaking it in just the right way to get the full power.

What is marvelous about this life balancing technique of vagus nerve stimulation is that it doesn't have to cost you a cent. With most cases being something that you can stimulate your nerve with at home and only a few that require a vagus nerve stimulator, it can put the power into your own hands and allow for a better quality of life overall.

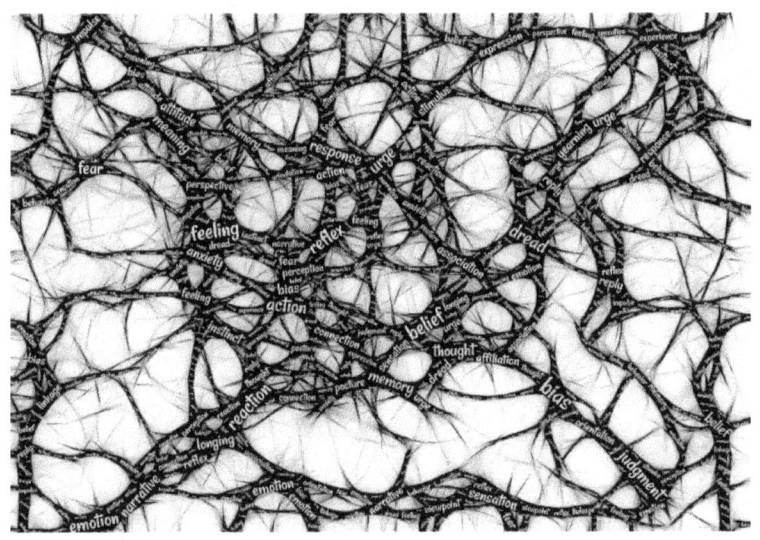

www.ingramcontent.com/pod-product-compliance
Lightning Source LLC
Chambersburg PA
CBHW071350210526
45465CB00001B/50